Contents

Preface

The graying of America . . . We are undoubtedly getting older. A person doesn't wake up one morning and look into the mirror and say, "You look old!" Aging is a gradual process that affects everyone; some at a faster rate than others.

Aging is something that no one can escape. And, as we age, we develop medical problems associated with growing old. EMT and paramedic programs have begun to recognize that the population of older adults is increasing and that training is needed to provide quality care for older individuals. Recognizing a weakness is the first step in correcting it.

This textbook is written to give the emergency care professional insight into the changes that occur as we age and the special problems experienced by older adults. It is written at the EMT-Intermediate level and above; however, all EMS professionals can glean important information from the material. Throughout the text we refer to the "prehospital care provider" (PHCP). This is a generic reference, and it applies to all levels of prehospital care personnel, including the first responder, EMT, EMT-Intermediate, paramedic, and mobile intensive care nurse.

The chapters of this book are organized to give the prehospital care provider information in a systematic approach—from the physical and emotional changes with growing old to medical emergencies. Additionally, a chapter is dedicated to the terminally ill patient.

Here is a summary of the chapters in this textbook.

CHAPTER 1: INTRODUCTION

This chapter discusses the graying of the U.S. population. Based on population measures from the U.S. Census Bureau, it is evident that, as a whole, the population of the United States is getting older. The chapter also addresses what impact this aging trend will have on the provision of emergency medical services to the community, especially in light of the federally mandated "Prudent Layperson Standard" covering emergencies.

CHAPTER 2: PHYSIOLOGICAL CHANGES WITH AGING

This chapter discusses the physical changes that occur as we age. Without question, the skin thins and becomes wrinkled, and the hair turns gray. But, there are many more other changes that occur. Each organ system is affected, and each system is discussed in a concise, easy-to-understand manner.

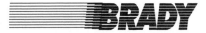

Geriatric Prehospital Care

Robert G. Nixon, BA, EMT-P
Life Care Medical Training

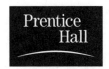

Prentice Hall

Upper Saddle River, New Jersey 07458

Library of Congress Cataloging-in-Publication Data

Nixon, Robert G.
  Geriatric prehospital care / Robert G. Nixon.—1st ed.
    p. cm.
  Includes index.
  ISBN 0-13-018682-1 (alk. paper)
  1. Medical emergencies. 2. Critical care medicine. 3. Geriatrics. I. Title.
[DNLM: 1. Emergencies—Aged. 2. Emergency Medical Services—Aged. 3. Emergency
Treatment—methods. 4. Geriatrics. WB 105 N736g 2002]
RC952.5 .N55 2002
618.97'6025—dc21

2001059334

Unless otherwise indicated all photos are provided by the author.

Publisher: *Julie Levin Alexander*
Assistant to Publisher: *Regina Bruno*
Senior Acquisitions Editor: *Katrin Beacom*
Editorial Assistant: *Kierra Kashickey*
Marketing Manager: *Tiffany Price*
Director of Production and Manufacturing: *Bruce Johnson*
Managing Production Editor: *Patrick Walsh*
Manufacturing Buyer: *Pat Brown*
Production Liaison: *Julie Li*
Production Editor: *Jennifer Welsch*
Creative Director: *Cheryl Asherman*
Cover Design Coordinator: *Maria Guglielmo*
Cover Designer: *Gary J. Sella*
Cover Images: *Corbis Digital Stock/Photo Researchers,Inc.*
Composition: *BookMasters, Inc.*
Printing and Binding: *The Banta Company*

Pearson Education LTD.
Pearson Education Australia PTY, Limited
Pearson Education Singapore, Pte. Ltd.
Pearson Education North Asia Ltd.
Pearson Education Canada, Ltd.
Pearson Educación de Mexico, S.A. de C.V.
Pearson Education—Japan
Pearson Education Malaysia, Pte. Ltd.
Pearson Education, Upper Saddle River, New Jersey

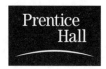

10 9 8 7 6 5 4 3 2 1
ISBN 0-13-018682-1

CHAPTER 3: PSYCHOSOCIAL CHANGES WITH AGING

Not only does the body change as it ages, but mental and emotional health can also be affected. Although mental prowess can be maintained until very late in life, there will be some slowing of mental processing. Depression is common in older adults, as is suicide ideation, especially in the older adult with chronic and debilitating conditions. Loneliness and isolation can also lead to alcohol or drug abuse. This chapter highlights the mental and emotional changes that may be evident in the older adult.

CHAPTER 4: PATIENT ASSESSMENT

The older patient can pose an assessment challenge to even the most seasoned EMS professional. This chapter presents information on patient assessment techniques that will help make the challenge less formidable. Information on communicating with the hearing or sight impaired is presented, along with tips on looking for more subtle information the older person may not admit or remember.

CHAPTER 5: ALZHEIMER'S DEMENTIA AND DELIRIUM

The media has frequently presented information on Alzheimer's dementia, paying particular attention to high-profile individuals who suffer from this devastating disease. But, Alzheimer's dementia is only one of many dementias. In addition, people may confuse delirium with dementia—an error based on misinformation. This chapter focuses on dementia and delirium, presenting information on each disorder. A mini mental status questionnaire is included to help in the assessment of impaired mental functioning.

CHAPTER 6: ELDER ABUSE—THE SILENT CRY

A new societal epidemic—elder abuse—has been identified. With an increasing number of older adults and an associated increase in the demand for care, stress on family caregivers has been tremendous. A side effect of this stress has been elder abuse. In many states, EMS professionals are legally obligated to report elder abuse to law enforcement or the appropriate state agency or face fines, imprisonment, or both. Chapter 6 discusses the five types of elder abuse. In addition to recognizing the types of abuse, the chapter also describes characteristics of the victim and the abuser. Finally, the chapter addresses guidelines for intervention and documentation of the abuse.

CHAPTER 7: PHARMACOLOGY IN THE OLDER POPULATION

Oftentimes, having a quality of life means taking prescription medications. Because of the aging process, many older adults take one or more medications for any number of medical conditions. Sometimes these medications can adversely affect the body. This chapter focuses on the hazards of medication use in the elderly. Beginning with basic pharmacology, the chapter discusses how a normal dose of an important medication can harm the older patient. This chapter also presents information on medications that should be used with caution or avoided by the geriatric patient. Finally, a section of the chapter is devoted to herbal supplements.

CHAPTER 8: MEDICAL EMERGENCIES: COMMON PROBLEMS SEEN IN THE ELDERLY

The older adult is prone to many of the same medical problems seen in the younger adult; however, there are conditions that are more frequently experienced by the geriatric patient. These conditions include falls, syncope, stroke, and others. Chapter 8 discusses the myriad of complaints the EMS provider may see when responding to a call involving the senior citizen.

CHAPTER 9: ACCIDENTAL INJURIES

The senior citizen is at a significant risk for falls and injuries caused by falling. Additionally, people with osteoporosis can sustain fractures with no apparent causative trauma. This chapter focuses on falls and injuries, including fractures, head injuries, burns, and carbon monoxide poisoning.

CHAPTER 10: FALL AND INJURY PREVENTION

Chapter 10 is dedicated to preventing the falls and injuries that so often lead to the premature death of many older adults. As a public service, many EMS agencies conduct in-home safety surveys to point out risks that could increase the chance of a fall or other accident.

CHAPTER 11: END-STAGE RENAL DISEASE

This chapter discusses a major chronic condition faced by many elderly patients—kidney failure and end-stage renal disease. The only treatment for this disease is dialysis or a kidney transplant. Although many patients have minimal complications associated with the condition, there are times when EMS will be called to care for a patient who is gravely ill from end-stage renal disease. An overview of dialysis is presented along with information on emergency care of the dialysis patient.

CHAPTER 12: THE TERMINALLY III PATIENT

Death and dying—something that the EMS professional sees all too frequently. Although our primary function is to delay or prevent premature death, there are some situations when the patient expects and even wants death. This chapter addresses the dying patient, including advanced directives and do not resuscitate orders. It also discusses the physical processes seen at the end of life. The information presented here is different from that found in many EMS textbooks.

CHAPTER 13: PUTTING IT ALL TOGETHER

Chapter 13 combines the information given in the preceding chapters and puts it all together in a general approach to the patient. From protecting the patient from the cold to properly applying the gurney straps, the EMS professional is given information to enhance their ability to care for other adults.

APPENDIX

The Appendix contains a listing of state agencies on aging and is current as of the date this book went to press. Additionally, sample forms for advanced directives, durable powers of attorney, and do not resuscitate orders are included for reference. The Appendix also contains a sample home safety checklist for use in injury prevention programs.

SPECIAL FEATURES

Objectives

Each chapter begins with a list of objectives that indicates what the reader can expect to accomplish by reading the chapter. These objectives can also be used as a self-test.

Words to Know

In addition to the objectives, each chapter has a list of Words to Know accompanied by each word's definition. Rather than going to the back of the book to look up terms in the glossary, important terms are listed at the start of each chapter.

Key Points

Throughout each chapter, key points are highlighted in boxes for easy reference. The reader can look for more detailed information on the topic within the text.

Sample Surveys

The text includes sample surveys that test for depression, mental acuity, and other clinical evaluations. This text also contains an in-home safety assessment that EMS providers can use to provide a valuable public service—education to reduce the risk of falls and injuries in the home.

On the Job

Most chapters have an On the Job feature that presents a situation commonly found in the field. These scenes can be discussed in class or in small study groups to reinforce the information in the chapter.

Acknowledgments

No textbook could be written without the assistance of a number of people working behind the scene. These people are the unsung heroes of any book and need to be thanked for their assistance in making the dream a reality.

I would like to extend a hearty thanks to the following people who participated in bringing this book to print. Dr. Chuck Stewart, Teena Foote, and Katja Thomas reviewed many chapters of the manuscript as they were being created and helped keep the text on track. Carol Anderson graciously volunteered to be a model in several pictures in the book, and Char Jacobs helped when extra hands were needed for a few of the shots. Thanks also go to Betty Sanchez with Walnut Creek Dialysis Center for allowing me to take pictures of the hemodialysis machine used in the chapter on End-State Renal Disease.

Finally, my thanks go to the staff at Brady including Judy Streger, Katrin Beacom, and Kierra Kashickey for initiating and following this book to completion. I sincerely appreciate your support and dedication to this project.

DEDICATION

This book is dedicated to my daughter, Jenn, who has made me proud of her accomplishments. Besides, she may one day have to choose my nursing home!

1

Introduction

At the end of this chapter, the reader will be able to:

1 Define a senior citizen as one who is at least 65 years of age.
2 Define the Baby Boomer generation as people born between 1946 and 1964.
3 State the average age of the United States population in 2000 as 35.3 years of age.
4 State the current average life expectancy of people living in the United States as 76 years of age.
5 Define the term "prudent layperson."
6 Explain how the prudent layperson standard applies to the definition of an emergency medical condition.
7 Explain how the prudent layperson standard applies to the definition of an urgent medical condition.
8 Discuss the effects of longevity on the future role of EMS.

Baby Boomer   A member of the generation of people born in the United States between the years of 1946 and 1964.

Dysfunction   Abnormal function of a body part or system.

Emergency medical condition   A condition that could, without immediate medical attention, result in jeopardizing the health of the person, cause serious impairment to bodily function, or cause serious dysfunction of any bodily organ.

Foley catheter   A tube inserted into the bladder and used to collect urine into a drainage bag. The catheter is held in place by an inflatable balloon.

Prudent layperson   A person who possesses an average knowledge of health and medicine.

Urgent medical condition   A condition for which medical care is necessary and immediately required, and for which any delay is not reasonable.

Health Care Financing Administration (HCFA)   Government agency responsible for overseeing Medicare.

Geriatrics. Elderly. Senior citizens. Older adults. These words often conjure up negative images that involve people who are unable to care for themselves; unable to bathe, feed, or dress themselves; or unable to communicate effectively. Often, we think of the elderly as confined to a wheelchair or hospital bed, stranded in a convalescent hospital or nursing home waiting for the inevitable—death. Although there are many older adults who exist in this manner, there are millions more leading active, healthy, and productive lives.

There is confusion as to what constitutes being 'old.' In a purely demographic context, turning 65 years of age places a person in the elderly population group. Yet, a person turning 50 qualifies for membership in AARP (formerly referred to as the American Association of Retired Persons). In some places, a person can qualify for "senior discounts" when they are 55 years of age. Thus, there is no set definition of being "old." In contrast, aging is a process that starts at birth and accelerates as we get older. Most references, including this text, assume that the age of 65 determines a person's passage into the geriatric age group.

THE POPULATION IS GETTING OLDER

According to Census Bureau estimates, the average age of the population of the United States is increasing. The Baby Boomer generation was born between the years 1946 and 1964, producing 78 million Americans. The number of births in this country since the Baby Boomer generation has not offset the advancing age of the Baby Boomers. In 1995, for example, the median age in the United States was 34.4 years. According to the 2000 census, the median age increased to 35.3 years. In 1996, the oldest of the Baby Boomers turned 50 and, by some estimates, one person turns 50 years of age every 8 minutes.

The number of people 65 years of age and older is also rapidly increasing. According to the Census Bureau, while the number of people under the age of 65 has tripled, the number of people over the age of 65 has increased 11-fold. At the turn of the twentieth century, the ratio of seniors to the general popula-

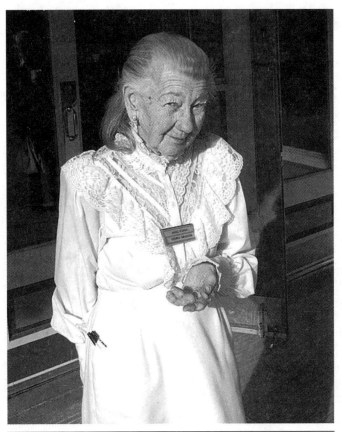

• FIGURE 1-1

Miss Edna, who only admits to being 80-something, is the Ambassador at the Gold Rush Casino in Cripple Creek, Colorado. The job keeps her very busy and she enjoys being active.

tion was one in 25. By the mid-1990s, that ratio had shrunk to one in eight. Population findings for the 2000 census show that, for the first time, the number of people over the age of 55 years will be nearly the same as the number of people under the age of 15. Because of declining fertility and increased longevity, by the middle of the twenty-first century the U.S. population could have one elderly person in every five Americans.

One of the most rapidly growing age groups is the over-85 population. In 1994, the number of over-85s was estimated at 3 million. The current census (2000) shows the number of over-85s is 4.2 million. If the current trend continues, that number is expected to rise to 19 million by the middle of the twenty-first century.

The primary reason for the increase in the age of the U.S. population is that we are living longer. During the early years of the United States, the average life expectancy was 35 years. That increased to 47 years of age by 1900 and 76 years of age by the early 1990s.

The reasons for our living longer include a better quality of life due to better economics and enhanced medical care, including earlier detection and better medical treatment of life-threatening diseases. Although cardiovascular disease is still the leading cause of death in the United States, mortality rates from cardiovascular disease have declined over the years due to advanced treatments. Additionally, although deaths due to cancer have increased for the elderly, newer treatments have prolonged the lives of many stricken with malignant or metastatic disease.

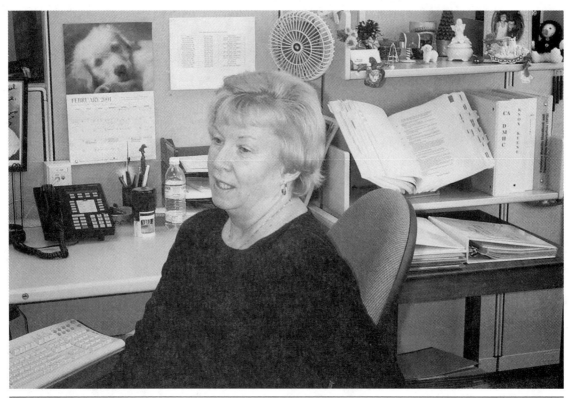

• FIGURE 1-2
Many older adults are actively employed.

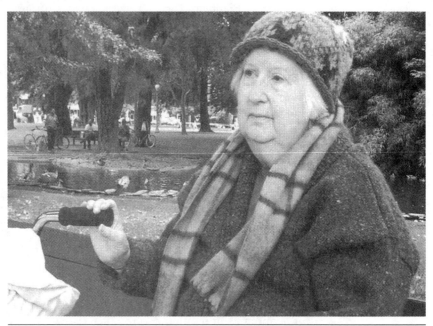

• FIGURE 1-3
The elderly enjoy a variety of activities such as walking.
Source: Courtesy Brady *MedEMT*, page 349.

HOUSING THE OLDER POPULATION

Because of special needs of the older adult, providing housing that meets those needs places a unique demand on the community. EMS may be called to a number of residences, all of which house aging adults with a myriad of needs.

Many older adults may choose not to relocate. Instead, they stay in the house where they have resided for many years. However, many are faced with a need to move. Considerations in making the decision to move to another residence include deteriorating neighborhood safety, proximity to their children, cost of home maintenance, increased physical or medical needs, transportation issues, and a desire for a new lifestyle.

Depending on their needs, the older adult has several options in choosing a residence. These options include:

- Retirement communities
- Continuing-care retirement communities
- Congregate senior housing
- Adult foster care
- Senior group homes
- Subsidized senior housing
- Assisted living facilities
- Board and care homes
- Skilled nursing facilities

Because prehospital care providers will be called to any one of these living facilities, it is important to be familiar with the different types of senior housing.

Retirement communities are age-restricted communities that state a minimum age for residency. Minimal assistance, if any, is provided. Some retirement communities are gated, meaning access is restricted and controlled through a guarded gate. This provides increased security for the older adult.

Continuing-care retirement communities are available for active seniors who want to live independently but have support for future medical care needs. As the person ages and medical needs increase, multiple levels of care are available within the community.

Congregate senior housing provides living facilities for older adults in separate apartments, yet also provides opportunities for shared activities, including meals and social events. Congregate housing may also provide varying levels of assistance such as assisted living, skilled nursing care, or Alzheimer's care.

Adult foster care is where a family opens their home to an older adult who rents a room within the home. Meals and other amenities are often provided in the foster care home. Some residential care may be provided depending on the senior citizen's needs.

Depending on the financial status of the older adult, subsidized housing may be necessary. Federal and state programs help pay for senior housing for those with low or moderate incomes. The residents live in separate apartments within the senior complex. If necessary, assistance with some chores, such as shopping or laundry, is provided.

If the older adult needs more care, assisted living facilities are also available. Assisted living is considered a general term and applies to those who live independently but occasionally need a small amount of help.

Board and care homes are group living arrangements for those who cannot live independently. An increased number of services are available, such as help with the activities of daily living, including bathing, dressing, eating, and toilet assistance.

Skilled nursing facilities are available for those in need of acute, intermediate, or long-term skilled nursing care. A few skilled nursing facilities provide specialized care for patients with Alzheimer's disease. Some skilled nursing facilities will also provide custodial care for those patients who do not need skilled nursing care.

THE EFFECTS OF LONGEVITY ON EMERGENCY SERVICES

Because of the effects of aging on the body, many older adults can suffer from multiple problems. Some of these problems, though chronic in nature, can worsen or become acute, requiring prehospital and emergency medical intervention. In the future, prehospital care providers will be faced with an increase in the number of responses to older adults calling for assistance, which may strain the local EMS agency and emergency department resources.

In some areas, an increase in the use of EMS and emergency department resources as a support service or walk-in clinic has been noted. The casual use of the emergency department for urgent and even routine medical care significantly stresses the system. Due to the economic demand on available resources, some health insurance carriers require their policyholders or members to call in and get permission to call an ambulance or visit the emergency department. This may change should a patient's bill of rights pass Congress. In that bill of rights, the definition of an emergency will be based on what is known as the "prudent layperson" standard. This standard was first adopted in the Balanced Budget Act of 1997 and currently affects all Medicare recipients.

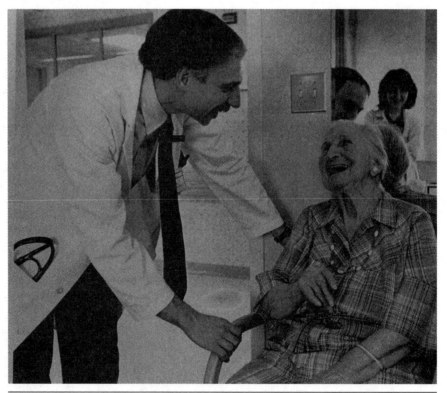

• FIGURE 1-4
Older adults may use the emergency department more often than other age groups.

Source: Picture courtesy of *Aging,* a magazine from the Administration on Aging, www.aoa. dhhs.gov/aoa/magimage/magimage.html.

In short, the prudent layperson standard states:

An emergency medical condition is a medical condition manifesting itself by acute symptoms of sufficient severity (including severe pain) such that a prudent layperson, who possesses an average knowledge of health and medicine, could reasonably expect the absence of immediate medical attention to result in (a) placing the health of the individual in jeopardy . . . , (b) serious impairment to bodily functions, or (c) serious dysfunction of any bodily organ or part.

An enhancement of the prudent layperson standard encompasses urgent medical conditions. An urgent medical condition is one for which care is medically necessary and immediately required because of unforeseen illness, injury, or condition, and it is not reasonable, given the circumstances, to delay care in order to obtain the services from the primary care physician.

In other words, if a person believes an emergency or urgent care situation exists, then it does exist, and emergency or urgent care will be provided. This holds true even if the medical condition is deemed not to have been an emergency or one that needed urgent attention. The standard is expected to increase the demand on EMS and emergency department facilities.

Older adults have placed calls to 9-1-1 dispatchers for a variety of non-emergent needs. For example, one 74-year-old man called 9-1-1 to have the paramedics remove his Foley catheter because it was irritating him. In another call, a woman requested 9-1-1 assistance to help her off the toilet. She had a progressive neurological disease and was temporarily unable to go from a sitting to a standing position. Her husband, a frail man, was unable to assist her but was able to call for help.

THE ROLE OF EMS

Our role as emergency care providers is changing. Although we must continue to provide professional and compassionate care for older adults in an emergent or urgent situation, we must face and adapt to the new challenges associated with the elderly population.

First, prehospital care providers must recognize the changing needs of the elderly patient. As we age, the body undergoes normal changes. These changes reduce our capacities and capabilities to function independently. The senior citizen may perceive any loss of function as the loss of independence. These changes in physiology will alter the way EMS provides emergency care. For example, medications must be carefully monitored for adverse effects and drug interactions. Dosages need to be altered due to the changes in drug metabolism and excretion. The authors of *Essentials of Clinical Geriatrics* very aptly state, "The least desirable outcome of medical care is a decrease in the patient's health as a result of contact with the care system. In some cases, there is a real risk that untoward consequences of treatment may worsen a patient's health."

Second, we in EMS need to be aware of available community resources that can assist in the care of the elderly. Statistics have shown that whereas older men are typically married, the elderly woman often lives alone. Frequently, EMS providers respond to calls in the middle of the night to attend to the "little old lonely lady" who is primarily seeking attention and assurance that she is fine. By introducing the lonely person to some available resources (e.g., community outreach programs, locations of nearby senior centers, etc.), the frequency of late-night calls for attention might be reduced.

Finally, EMS providers must become acutely aware of the increased potential for elder abuse. As the population ages, its younger members will be increasingly called upon to care for the elderly. Long-term care facilities are expensive, and, under the Balanced Budget Act of 1997, the Health Care Financing Administration (HCFA) has curtailed funding of home healthcare services. The burden for caring for the elderly will continue to shift onto family members who, with stresses of their own, may be unable or unwilling to provide quality care for their aging parents. Internal and external stresses can lead to physical and other forms of elder abuse. If abuse is suspected, prehospital care providers must report their suspicions to the appropriate state or local agencies.

SUMMARY

The population in the United States is getting older. The aging process brings physical and psychological changes that may require prompt intervention by prehospital care providers. Our role in prehospital care is constantly changing, and will continue to do so as we meet the challenges presented by the older population.

The assessment and care of the older adult means that prehospital care providers must possess specialized information about the aging process and the ability to recognize the signs and symptoms of geriatric emergencies. However, recognizing the special needs of the elderly is only a small aspect of prehospital care of the senior citizen. We must also be able to provide emergency care that will alleviate the emergency and, when possible, begin the process of restoring function and independence to the patient.

ON THE JOB

Think about the number of calls you answer in a 24-hour period. How many of the calls are for pediatric patients? How many are for adults aged 18–50? How many are for adults aged 50–64? How many of the calls are for patients over the age of 65? Older adults need and seek medical help far more often than younger patients. The elderly also need more care, have multiple medical problems, and take more medications, making prehospital care and assessment a tremendous challenge.

2

Physiological Changes with Aging

Alveoli   Air sacs in the lung where oxygen-carbon dioxide exchange takes place.

Arcus senilis   Grayish arc or ring around the outer edge of the iris caused by calcium and cholesterol deposits. Does not affect sight.

Arteriosclerosis   Hardening of the arteries.

Atherosclerosis   Narrowing of the artery by a deposit of plaque.

Baroreceptors   Pressure sensors in the carotid artery of the neck and aorta that monitor blood pressure.

Cardiac output   The amount of blood the heart pumps per heart beat (contraction).

Cataract   A clouding of the lens of the eye that reduces vision.

Collagen   A fibrous protein that makes up the white structures of the skin and provides support for other tissues in the body.

Dehydration   Excessive loss of body water.

Dorsalis pedis pulse   Pulse found on the top of the foot behind the third toe. The pulse is created when blood flows through the dorsalis pedis artery.

Electrical conduction system   A pathway through the heart through which the heart's electrical current travels.

Floaters   Opaque parts of the fluid in the back of the eye that float across the visual field.

Heat stroke   A condition caused by excessively high body temperature brought on by exposure to a hot environment.

Hypercapnia   Excessive carbon dioxide levels in the arterial blood.

Hypertension   High blood pressure.

Hypothalamus   An area of the brain that controls many of the involuntary functions of the body, including sleep, hunger, thirst, and temperature control.

Hypothermia   Low body temperature.

Hypoxia   Abnormally low oxygen levels in the arterial blood.

Intestinal motility   Spontaneous movement within the intestines.

Iris   The colored portion of the eye that controls the size of the pupil.

Kyphosis   Abnormal curvature of the upper spine. Also known as hunchback.

Macular degeneration   Deterioration of the focal point of the eye. It causes low vision.

Neuropathy   Deterioration of peripheral nerves, possibly leading to the loss of sensation or numbness in the affected area.

Osteoporosis   Loss of bone mass caused by a loss of calcium from the bone.

Peristalsis   Wave-like contraction found in the intestines that propels digesting food through the gastrointestinal system.

Retina   The lining of the back of the eye where light-sensitive neurons sense light and transmit it to the brain by way of the optic nerve.

Retinal artery occlusion   Blockage of one of the arteries in the retina. It can lead to blindness.

Retinal vein occlusion   Blockage of one of the veins in the retina of the eye. It can lead to blindness or low vision.

Skin turgor   A reflection of the skin's elasticity and hydration.

With normal aging, the body changes. Most people rarely notice these changes because they are subtle. A person does not awaken one day to find him- or herself old with wrinkled skin and gray hair. Some of these normal changes can pose problems in the assessment and treatment of the acutely ill older adult. Along with the normal changes that accompany aging, there may be some pathological changes that can contribute to the early demise of the patient.

EMS personnel need to recognize the normal aging process so that they can differentiate what is normal from what is abnormal. Recognizing the normal changes associated with aging will assist in the assessment of the overall condition of the geriatric patient, helping the prehospital care provider to probe for serious, underlying conditions that may be hidden.

The geriatric patient is more prone to serious cardiac and respiratory illnesses. For example, pneumonia is common in elderly patients and can be fatal. Serious illness can be devastating to the older adult because the body has less ability to compensate. Although an older person may have no cardiac or respiratory problems at rest, they may become short of breath with minimal exertion. In the event of an infectious disease, the elderly patient may not develop fever to help thwart the infection. Or, in the event of an accident, the heart rate cannot adjust as quickly to compensate for a decrease in blood pressure.

The aging process can lead to general deterioration and a multitude of health concerns. Prehospital care providers frequently encounter older patients who have more than one chronic condition. Consider, for example, the older patient with a history of adult-onset diabetes, emphysema, and heart disease.

Finally, the aging process may predispose a patient to sustain a serious injury after what appears to be minor trauma. For example, an elderly woman with osteoporosis could sustain a fractured hip by simply turning or twisting her legs while standing at the kitchen counter.

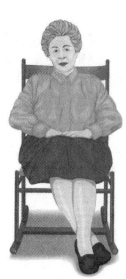

Decreased mentation
Depression common
May resist efforts to help

Decreased vision
Decreased hearing

Decreased cardiac output
Decreased heart rate
Irregular heart rhythm
Increased blood pressure

Osteoporosis common
Fractures occur more easily
Osteoarthritis common
Muscle mass decreased
Mobility decreased

Skin is thinner
Skin can tear easily
Skin bruises easily
Skin turgor delayed

Decreased elasticity of airways
Decreased cough ability
Increased resistance in chest
Decreased tidal volume

• FIGURE 2-1
Aging brings changes in the body.
Source: Courtesy Brady Prehospital Emergency Care, p. 221.

The purpose of this chapter is to familiarize the prehospital care provider with the normal changes associated with aging. Most organ systems will be discussed and examples of what might be seen in the normal older patient will be presented.

OVERALL APPEARANCE

The elderly patient generally appears shorter in stature and may be stooped due to bone loss. Deterioration in the thoracic spine may cause a hunchback appearance (kyphosis). The patient may appear abnormally thin due to loss of muscle mass and perhaps dehydration. The eyes may appear sunken due to weight loss.

THE SKIN

With increasing age, the skin thins and wrinkles begin to appear. Additionally, the junction of the epidermis and dermis flattens and the epidermis tends to separate from the dermis. Because of these changes, the skin becomes more permeable, allowing infections to develop more easily.

As the skin ages, the elasticity of the skin decreases as the dermis thins and collagen support is lost. This loss of elasticity contributes to wrinkling of the skin, hastening sun damage, and results in a higher susceptibility for bruising from minor trauma. Healing of superficial wounds may also take longer in the elderly patient.

When the skin becomes thin and less elastic, the process of checking for skin turgor and adequate hydration is changed. To assess hydration in the average-aged adult, the prehospital care provider gently pinches the skin on the back of the hand, creating a slight tent. Upon releasing the skin, it should immediately return to its normal state when hydration is adequate. In the elderly patient, the skin on the back of the hand has lost its resiliency and will remain tented even in the presence of adequate hydration. To properly assess skin turgor in an older adult, gently tent the skin on the older adult's cheek, chest, or abdomen.

In the elderly patient, support for the blood vessels in the skin decreases. Without vessel support and protection, a minor bump could result in bruising and bleeding. Further, as vessel support decreases, the number of cutaneous blood vessels decreases. Circulation to the skin is reduced, ultimately impairing heat loss, increasing the chance of pressure sores (decubitus ulcers), and prolonging wound healing.

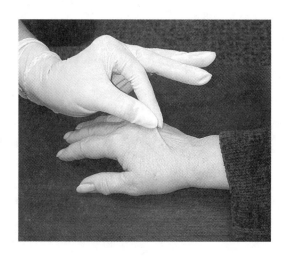

• FIGURE 2-2A
Tenting the skin on the back of the hand to assess turgor is fine in the younger adult. In the older adult, loss of elasticity may give a false positive result.

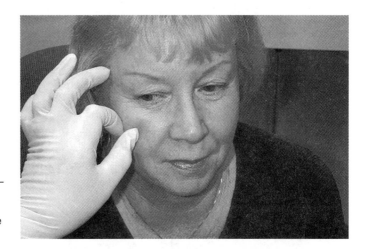

• FIGURE 2-2B
Instead of using the skin on the back of the hand, use the skin on the cheek.

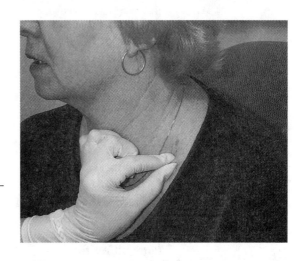

• FIGURE 2-2C
The skin on the upper chest can also be used to assess skin turgor.

The sweat and oil glands of the skin also deteriorate as a person ages, decreasing their ability to dissipate heat. Heat stroke in the elderly is a significant problem during the summer months. Another effect of this deterioration is that the skin tends to be dryer and more easily irritated due to the lack of sweat and oil.

KEY POINT

Changes in the skin increase the risk of heat-related illness in the elderly.

The skin's specialized nerve sensors decrease in number and become distorted as a person ages. Such a change could impair the geriatric patient's sensory perception, and they might not be able to differentiate hot from cold as easily as when they were younger. Perception of pain can also be altered.

KEY POINT

Changes in the nerves in the skin can alter the older person's ability to sense pain or differentiate between hot and cold.

Another component of the integumentary system affected by the aging process is the hair. With aging, the hair thins. In men, a receding hairline and baldness are common. Hair loss has a number of causes. With increasing age, the number of hair follicles decreases, resulting in thinner hair. Additionally, medications and medical conditions also lead to hair loss.

Gray hair develops when the pigment-producing cells (melanocytes) in the hair follicles stop working. Without this pigment called melanin, a strand of hair becomes transparent. Its gray color is attributed to the cells that make up the hair. These changes in physical appearance can impact self-image and contribute to depression.

CARDIOVASCULAR SYSTEM

The heart and blood vessels undergo normal changes with aging. These changes increase the risk of disease and may change the nature of the onset of illness. Ultimately, these changes can affect the overall treatment and progression of cardiovascular disease. There are many factors that affect the cardiovascular system over time. Smoking, hypertension, a sedentary lifestyle, and poor or inappropriate diet all contribute to early deterioration of the cardiovascular system.

The heart is affected by the aging process in many ways. The musculature may remain unchanged or it may atrophy or enlarge depending on the factors mentioned previously. In a healthy older adult, the blood flow out of the heart (cardiac output) may not be affected by age. However, in an unhealthy older adult, the heart's ability to pump effectively can be reduced. If the amount of blood pumped from the heart is decreased, oxygenation of the vital organs and peripheral tissues is significantly affected.

The maximum heart rate decreases as age increases. The maximum heart rate is determined by subtracting a person's age from 220 beats per minute. Therefore, a 20-year-old adult has a maximum heart rate of 200 beats per minute, whereas a 70-year-old adult has a maximum heart rate of 150 beats per minute. At rest, this difference is not noticeable. With exercise or any physical demand on the heart for additional output, the difference in maximum heart rate can be substantial.

The heart rate can be affected by stimuli from receptors that monitor the blood pressure. These receptors, called baroreceptors, are located in the carotid

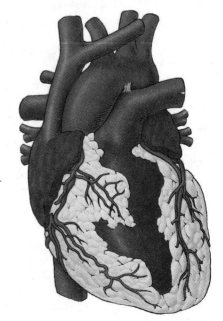

• FIGURE 2-3
Decreased heart rate and force of contraction are common as a person ages. The heart's conduction system also deteriorates leading changes in the ECG.
Source: Courtesy of Brady, *MedEMT*, p. 121.

arteries in the neck and in the aorta. When the blood pressure increases or decreases, these sensors will cause an opposite response in the heart rate. In the younger adult, an increase or decrease of 1 mm mercury (Hg) in blood pressure causes a one beat per minute decrease or increase in heart rate. This same ratio is not typical in the elderly patient, especially those on multiple medications. In the older adult, for every 1 mm Hg change in blood pressure, the heart rate may change by one-half a beat per minute. Thus, for an older adult in shock, the heart rate may not increase significantly, even in the presence of low blood pressure.

The heart is controlled by electrical impulses traveling through the body's electrical conduction system. Impulses normally begin at the sinoatrial node in the upper-right atrium and travel over a predetermined pathway to the ventricles. With aging, the electrical conduction system can deteriorate. The elderly patient may experience abnormalities in heart rhythm that could be considered "normal" for that person. However, some abnormalities are pathologic and require intervention. If an irregular heartbeat is noted on examination, ask the patient if that irregularity is normal for them.

KEY POINT

The heart's pumping ability can deteriorate due to changes in heart rate, force of contraction, and rhythm. This could lead to fainting, mental confusion, fatigue, and other serious problems.

Aging changes the flow of blood through the blood vessels. Atherosclerosis and arteriosclerosis are common conditions that lead to decreased blood flow through the arteries, resulting in a reduction in tissue oxygenation. Assessment of peripheral blood flow may be difficult. For example, the dorsalis pedis pulse on the foot may be hard to find. Hardening of the arteries may also increase the patient's blood pressure. Hypertension is fairly common in elderly patients. Even though it is common in the elderly, hypertension is still considered a pathologic condition.

KEY POINT

Arteriosclerosis and atherosclerosis reduce blood flow to the organs and decrease oxygenation of vital tissues. They can also lead to hypertension.

Additionally, hardening of the arteries affects the immune system, as the immune system cannot detect and respond to infectious agents if tissue perfusion has been reduced.

RESPIRATORY SYSTEM

Aging affects the respiratory system in two ways. First, aging affects the function of the lung, including ventilation and the exchange of oxygen and carbon dioxide. Second, aging impairs the ability of the lungs to protect themselves against illness.

As a person ages, the lungs and chest wall change. The lungs lose elasticity, which impairs the lungs' ability to recoil or return to normal size after

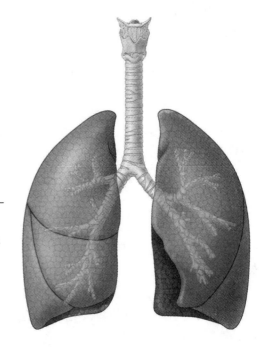

• FIGURE 2-4
Changes in the respiratory
system can lead to shortness
of breath on minimal exertion. Allow the older adult
to 'catch' the breath as
needed.
Source: Courtesy of Brady,
MedEMT, p. 110i.

inhalation. The exact mechanism for this change in elasticity is not fully understood. The chest wall stiffens, possibly as a result of calcification of the ribs
where they join the sternum or spine. The end result of this stiffening is the trapping of air within the alveoli, as noted by a slight increase in total lung capacity
and a larger increase in other lung volumes such as functional residual capacity
(air remaining after normal exhalation) and residual volume (air remaining after
forceful exhalation). Although most prehospital care providers are familiar with
the barrel chest found in patients with chronic obstructive pulmonary disease
(COPD), it is very possible to find a barrel chest in a patient without COPD.

Due to the loss of elasticity of the lung and, perhaps, loss of bronchial muscle
tone, airflow out of the lungs is also impaired. This, too, increases air trapping.

In addition to impairments in getting air into the lungs, there is also a reduction in the ability to diffuse oxygen and carbon dioxide. The aging process
primarily affects oxygen-carbon dioxide exchange in the alveoli due to loss of
alveolar tissue and a thickening of some of the tiny air sacs. An additional effect of aging is the decreased ability of oxygen to combine with available blood.

Along with pulmonary function changes, the older adult also experiences
changes in breathing control. For example, the effects of hypoxia on the rate and
depth of ventilation are reduced. The healthy older patient's response to hypoxia
is about half that of a 22-year-old. Similarly, when the level of carbon dioxide in
the blood is increased (hypercapnia), healthy younger adults will quickly double
the rate and depth of breathing. In the healthy senior citizen, this response is reduced by over 40 percent. Keep in mind, these reductions are seen in the healthy
older adult. In those geriatric patients with underlying respiratory diseases such
as emphysema or chronic bronchitis, the effects are more pronounced.

KEY POINT

The elasticity of the lungs changes with age, affecting oxygen-carbon dioxide exchange. Hypoxia can result, leading to shortness of breath, fainting,
or other problems.

The older adult is more susceptible to respiratory diseases due to a decrease in the lungs' ability to protect themselves. With increasing age, there is a decreased cough reflex. If the elderly patient cannot reflexively cough, there is an increased risk of aspiration and pneumonia. Further, the normal defense mechanism of mucus and cilia is also affected by advancing age. In the average-aged adult, mucus traps foreign particles, and the cilia move the mucus upward along the tracheobronchial tree. With a cough, the mucus and debris are expelled from the airways. This normal mechanism deteriorates with age, which could lead to chronic bronchitis or other pulmonary inflammation.

KEY POINT

Changes in the airways and lungs that occur with aging can make the older adult more susceptible to infections such as pneumonia.

Not only do the initial defenses of the respiratory system deteriorate, but the immune system in the lungs also loses function. If the patient cannot clear secretions from the airways and the immune system does not respond adequately, the chance of severe respiratory illness is significantly increased.

MUSCULOSKELETAL SYSTEM

As mentioned at the beginning of this chapter, the senior citizen experiences a loss of body weight as well as a loss of bone structure. Perhaps because of decreased nutrition, muscle mass deteriorates and the elderly person loses body weight. Occasionally, the older adult may appear emaciated.

With the loss of muscle mass, the elderly person has little ability to control heat loss or gain. With heat loss, the average-aged adult will begin to shiver to generate additional body heat. Because there is reduced muscle mass, the elderly do not shiver. Hypothermia can be pronounced in the senior citizen even in the absence of extremely cold temperatures and shivering.

KEY POINT

Loss of muscle mass can increase the risk for hypothermia.

Weaker muscles also impair the older person's ability to move and provide self-care. Loss of muscle mass also increases the risk of injury from falls. The elderly also have an increased tendency to drop things. If an older adult is impaired, they may not be able to adequately hydrate or feed themselves. This aggravates the weight loss.

Osteoporosis is a disease that affects both older men and women. Osteoporosis is defined as a bone disorder resulting in a gradual loss of bone mass. With the loss of bone mass, there is an increased likelihood of fractures, even after a seemingly minor trauma. Although a fall or lifting can precipitate the fracture, other causes of fractures include coughing, turning over in bed, or twisting the lower body. Typical fracture sites include the spine, wrist, and hip. The patient is often unaware of the disease until a fracture occurs. Women have a higher incidence of osteoporosis than men, and are at a greater risk for a hip fracture. Statistics show that one in three women will fracture a hip during her lifetime compared with one in eight men.

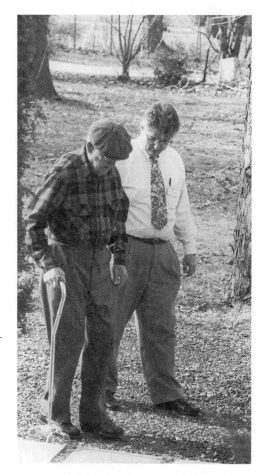

• FIGURE 2-5
Changes in the musculo-
skeletal system may require
the use of a cane while
walking.
Source: From *Aging*, a magazine
of the Administration on Aging.
www.aoa.dhhs.gov/aoa/
magimage/magimage.html.

KEY POINT

Osteoporosis is a significant problem that places the older adult at an increased risk for falls or spontaneous fractures.

NERVOUS SYSTEM

The central and peripheral nervous systems are affected by aging. The brain decreases in size and the number of cells in the cerebral cortex decreases. With advancing age, the senior citizen may have a slower-than-normal response to
verbal and physical stimuli. It may take a few moments longer to process in-
coming information. Thus, the elderly patient should be questioned more
slowly to accommodate for the delay in response. Not only will the elderly patient's verbal responses be slower, their psychomotor skills will also be slower.
The completion of a task for an elderly patient may take considerably more time,
so expect delays. For example, asking the older adult to gather belongings for
the trip to the hospital may result in prolonged on-scene time.

KEY POINT

Mental function can slow with age. After asking a question, wait for the
response.

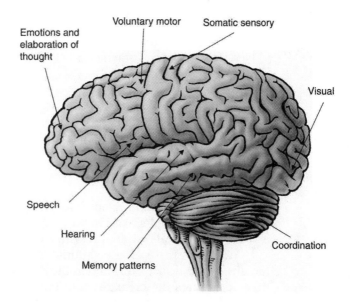

Emotions and elaboration of thought · Voluntary motor · Somatic sensory · Visual · Speech · Hearing · Memory patterns · Coordination

• FIGURE 2-6

Functional areas of the brain.

Source: Courtesy of Brady, *MedEMT*, p. 133.

As the brain ages, some of the physiological functions of the brain deteriorate. Control of the rate and depth of breathing and the response of the heart rate to blood pressure changes (discussed earlier) are two of the associated changes. Control of hunger and thirst are also regulated in the brain. With advancing age, the hypothalamus may not respond to the need for fluid or nutrition. A senior may become dehydrated or malnourished simply because they do not sense thirst or hunger.

Temperature regulation is also controlled by the hypothalamus. In the average aged adult, sensors along the spine send signals to the brain when the body is cooling or overheating. The body's response is to generate heat or dissipate it as needed. The aging process alters this response. In some elderly persons, the ambient temperature needs to change by at least 10°F in order for the person's body to detect a change.

KEY POINT

Deteriorating brain function can reduce the body's response to thirst, hunger, heat, and cold.

The aging process also affects the peripheral nerves. As mentioned in the discussion of the skin, with aging, the nerve sensors decrease in number and can become distorted. There may be a significant decrease in the patient's ability to sense touch and vibration. Altered or absent sensory perception can affect the person's ability to respond to physical stimuli. If the sensory nerves are altered, sensory reflexes can also be altered. If a person cannot sense heat or pain, they may not reflexively withdraw from heat or fire and could sustain a serious burn. Conversely, overstimulation of senses may produce an exaggeration of pain.

Changes in the peripheral nervous system also affect the older person's ability to sense movement or change in position (proprioception). This decreased ability to sense postural changes can increase the incidence of falling.

Patients with diabetes mellitus may have an exacerbated deterioration of these pain sensors. Peripheral neuropathy is common among diabetics; many cannot feel pain, and some have complained of numbness of the extremities.

GASTROINTESTINAL SYSTEM

As the gastrointestinal system ages, the patient may experience a drop in the amount of saliva, a decrease in the amount of hydrochloric acid in the stomach, and altered peristalsis in the intestines.

With a decrease in saliva, initial stages of digestion may be impaired. This impairment may also continue in the stomach, where a decrease in hydrochloric acid hinders the breakdown of ingested foods. It should be noted that although hydrochloric acid decreases, the incidence of ulcer disease is not affected. In addition, the diminished ability of the gastrointestinal system to absorb certain nutrients may impair nutrition. All of these factors can contribute to loss of muscle and bone, along with generalized wasting.

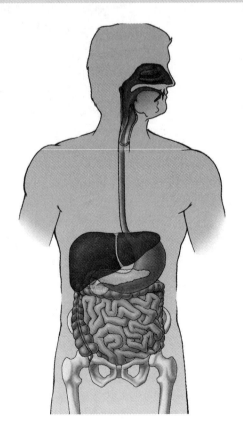

• FIGURE 2-7
Changes in the digestive system can impair nutrition and hydration.
Source: Courtesy of Brady, *MedEMT*, p. 1.

Intestinal motility can be altered by a number of factors, and generally results in constipation. If peristalsis of the intestines is slowed due to advancing age, inactivity, medications, or disease processes, the senior may require laxatives. Excessive use of laxatives can lead to dehydration and electrolyte imbalances.

Although not directly associated with the absorption of nutrients in the digestive system, intake of food can be impaired by dental problems such as poor or missing teeth, as well as improperly fitting dentures. Insufficient food intake will also contribute to wasting.

LIVER AND KIDNEYS

The effect of the aging process on the liver and kidneys is important from an EMS standpoint with regards to medications, either those the patient takes on his or her own or those we in EMS may administer at the scene and en route to the hospital.

The liver is responsible for metabolizing many medications and, with advancing age, its metabolic function slows. Blood flow to and through the liver is decreased, therefore some medications are not metabolized as rapidly. Because of this, the half-life of some medications may be substantially increased, along with their intended as well as adverse effects.

KEY POINT

Decreased liver function impairs the metabolism of drugs. A dose that is normal in the young adult could be toxic in the elderly patient.

With age, blood flow to the kidneys decreases, as does the filtration rate of the blood. For medications excreted through the kidney, the excretion rate may be significantly delayed, prolonging the effects of the medication.

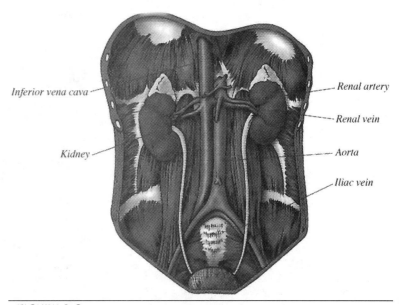

Inferior vena cava

Kidney

Renal artery

Renal vein

Aorta

Iliac vein

• FIGURE 2-8
With age the kidney function deteriorates.
Source: Courtesy of Brady, *MedEMT*, p. 127.

The senses also change with age. Sight and hearing will sustain varying degrees of loss and can impair the senior's ability to function independently. A loss or decrease in a patient's vision or hearing may also impact patient assessment.

As a person ages, changes in the inner ear may result in a loss of the ability to hear certain sound frequencies. Higher frequencies are the initial ones to be lost. With more advanced hearing loss, the ability to discriminate various pitches may also be affected. Extraneous noise can interfere with the patient's ability to distinguish the voice of the prehospital care provider and to answer questions appropriately. Communications with the elderly patient can become difficult at best. Some helpful tips on establishing effective communications with the hearing-impaired older adult will be discussed in the chapter on patient assessment.

Sight can be affected by aging. When initially examining the eyes, the prehospital care provider may note a grayish arc or ring at the top of the iris. This is known as the arcus senilis, and is caused by calcium and cholesterol deposits. The arcus senilis generally has no significant effect on patient assessment or on vision.

The iris regulates the size of the pupil and its reaction to light. As a person ages, the musculature changes and the pupil becomes smaller, reacting to light more sluggishly. For example, the pupil may dilate more slowly in the dark or constrict more slowly in bright light. Accommodation, or the response of the opposite eye when one eye is stimulated with light, is also slower. Accommodation also applies to the ability of the eyes to focus. Age-related changes reduce the eyes' abilities to focus, and a person's sight can be diminished. The patient's vision may be hampered by sudden changes in lighting until the iris can adjust.

KEY POINT

Pupillary response to light slows with age. A sluggish response to light may be normal.

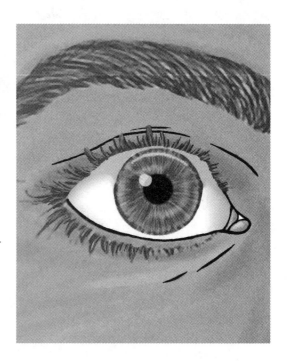

• FIGURE 2-9
Arcus senilis is a gray arch at the top or bottom of the eye. It has no effect on vision.
Source: Courtesy of Brady, *MedEMT*, p. 110.

A common complaint as we age is the reduced ability to clearly see things that are close. It seems that the arms are just too short to allow focusing when reading. The loss of elasticity in the lens of the eye due to aging tends to cause farsightedness. This condition is known as presbyopia. Without glasses, the ability to read the print on medication bottles can be impaired, resulting in medication errors.

A number of older adults receive treatment for glaucoma, an abnormal condition characterized by high pressure within the eye. Patients with chronic glaucoma use eye drops to reduce pressure in the eyes. Over time, and especially without treatment, the patient may lose peripheral vision. The patient may also complain of a dull pain in the affected eye, along with headache and blurring of vision.

The retina also changes with age. Although most prehospital care providers will not assess visual acuity, it is important to be aware of the changes in vision that can occur with aging. A very common problem found in the elderly population is age-related macular degeneration. It is generally a slow process during which the focal point on the retina (macula) deteriorates. The patient gradually complains of loss of vision and sees wavy vertical and horizontal lines rather than straight lines. Other problems associated with the retina that affect visual acuity include retinal detachment and occlusion of the retinal artery or retinal vein. These conditions need a prompt referral to an ophthalmologist.

KEY POINT

Sudden loss of vision in one eye could be due to an occluded artery or vein or a detached retina. Any sudden loss of vision is an emergency.

In addition to changes in the retina, there are other changes associated with the eye that prehospital care providers may encounter. These conditions include cataracts, dry eye, foreign-body sensation, and floaters.

A cataract is the clouding of the lens. With advancing age, the lens, through which all light must pass to reach the retina, becomes opaque. It appears as a graying of the lens and may affect visual acuity by increasing glare from bright lights.

KEY POINT

A cataract clouds the lens and makes sight similar to looking through fog.

Dry eye is a condition that results from a decrease in tear production. The elderly patient may also complain of the existence of a foreign body on the surface of the eye that continually causes irritation. Upon close examination, no foreign body can be found.

Floaters are pieces of solidified vitreous humor, the gel-like substance that fills the rear chamber of the eye. These opacities float freely in the remaining gel and occasionally cross the line of sight. Initially, floaters can be irritating, but are usually insignificant. However, multiple floaters accompanied the appearance of flashing lights in the peripheral visual field could signal retinal detachment.

By the age of 70, poor vision is common. Take additional time to assess the patient and determine related complaints. Taking time to explain what is happening to the patient with low vision can enhance the overall care of the older adult.

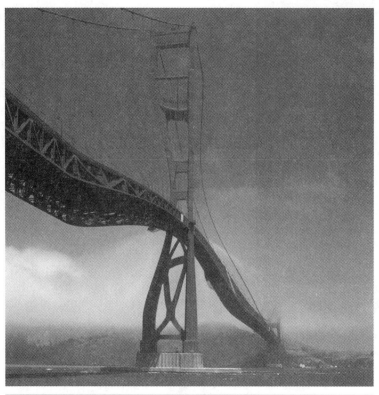

• FIGURE 2-10
Macular degeneration and retinal vessel occlusion can cause visual distortion.

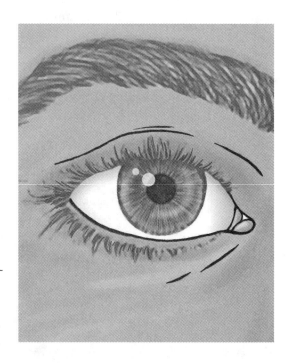

• FIGURE 2-11
A cloudy lens indicates a cataract.

Source: Courtesy of Brady *Paramedic Emergency Care*, p. 457.

SUMMARY

This chapter has focused on the physical changes that occur with aging. Every person undergoes these changes. Some people experience these changes sooner than others. Many of these changes are considered normal. Aging affects various organ

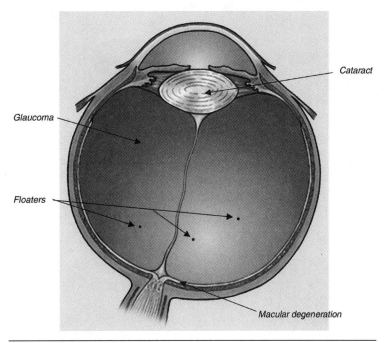

• FIGURE 2-12

Changes in the eye with aging can lead to vision impairment.

Source: Courtesy of Brady *Paramedic Emergency Care,* p. 457.

systems and may impair the older adult's normal functioning. These changes can also hinder the prehospital care provider's assessment of the elderly patient. The skin dries and wrinkles, the heart beats more slowly, the rate and depth of breathing diminish, and the nervous system slows. These changes are normal and need no intervention by EMS. When these normal changes accompany serious disease processes, immediate intervention can make the difference between returning the elderly patient to an acceptable level of functioning or watching the patient succumb to the ravages of time.

By understanding the normal changes associated with aging, as well as knowing about the pathology of the diseases encountered in the prehospital setting, the prehospital care provider can provide prompt and thorough assessment and care to the senior citizen in distress.

ON THE JOB

You receive a call to a private residence where you are greeted by an elderly man who tells you his wife is in the bathroom. You arrive at the bathroom door and find an older woman sitting on the toilet. In front of her is her walker. She looks over to you and says, "I'm stuck." In assessing the woman you learn that she has a progressive neuromuscular disease and that she occasionally is unable to go from sitting to standing. She says that her husband is too weak to help her up. Mrs. Jones asks, "I've been here for an hour, can you get me back to bed?" A quick check reveals no trauma, but you do notice a slightly irregular pulse that she claims is normal. What care and treatment should you offer Mrs. Jones?

3

Psychosocial Changes with Aging

OBJECTIVES

At the end of the chapter, the reader will be able to:

1 Discuss the effects of aging on mental capacity.

2 Discuss how some medical conditions, such as cardiovascular disease, can impair intellectual functioning.

3 Explain that abnormal behavior can be attributed to dementia or other organic causes.

4 List 12 risk factors for suicide in the elderly.

5 List nine signs or symptoms of depression.

6 List six risk factors for depression.

7 Describe how aging can increase the risk for depression.

8 Describe how prescription medications can cause the signs and symptoms of depression.

9 Explain that medical conditions are associated with depression.

10 Describe how a seemingly minor complaint can mask underlying depression.

11 Explain how the elderly patient's fear of the loss of independence can affect patient assessment and treatment.

12 Explain how the elderly patient's fear of death can affect patient assessment and treatment.

13 List the three types of antidepressants.

14 List two medications in each category of antidepressants.

15 List three types of elderly drinkers.

16 List two contributing factors to increased alcohol consumption in older adults.

17 State three reasons why the effects of alcohol are increased in the older adult.

WORDS TO KNOW

Anemia   Low number of red blood cells.

Chronic obstructive pulmonary disease (COPD)   A general description for emphysema and chronic bronchitis.

Delirium   Abnormal behavior that develops over a short time.

Dementia   Loss of cognitive functions over a period of time.

Depression   Altered mood with feelings of despair, sadness, and discouragement.

Hyperglycemia   Abnormally elevated blood sugar.

Hypoglycemia   Abnormally low blood sugar.

Hypoxia   Abnormally low oxygen levels in the arterial blood.

Insomnia   The perception of inadequate or unrestful sleep.

Osteoporosis   Loss of bone mass caused by a loss of calcium from the bone.

Palpitations   A heartbeat that is unusually fast or strong enough to make the person aware of the heartbeat.

Suicide gesture   An attempted suicide, but with the hope of being discovered and death prevented.

Suicide ideation   Frequent thoughts of suicide.

Transient ischemic attack (TIA)   A temporary block in the blood flow to an area of the brain. Mimics a stroke, but resolves within minutes.

In the previous chapter, we focused on the physical changes that everyone undergoes as they get older. There are also psychological changes that affect people during the later years of life. One of the primary psychological disorders associated with aging is depression. However, there are other psychological problems that prehospital care providers may encounter in the prehospital setting. This chapter will discuss some of the psychological effects of aging and examine the effects of aging on the geriatric patient's behavior. Please note that dementia and delirium are discussed in a separate chapter (Chapter 5).

EFFECTS OF AGING ON MENTAL FUNCTIONING

During the younger years, mental prowess, including math and verbal skills, increase over time until a person reaches 50 years of age. These skills then stabilize between the ages of 50 and 60. Some studies have cast doubt on the notion that, with age, mental capabilities deteriorate. Although men in their 70s and 80s may show a decline in some intellectual functions such as math, other intellectual functions, such as vocabulary, have been known to increase. In addition, the elderly maintain their ability to understand a given situation and can learn from experience. For example, an elderly woman who lives in a senior apartment complex was overheard saying, "Someone told me that I should go live in a nursing home. I told him to move in and let me know how it is. I take care of myself and don't need any help." The woman had recently celebrated her 103rd birthday!

However, some diseases do affect mental performance. Some studies have shown that men with cardiovascular disease have a significantly higher deterioration in intellectual functioning than those without, suggesting that factors other than normal aging affect mental capabilities. If a person shows significant mental deterioration, it may be caused by a pathological process rather than normal aging. Similarly, psychological disturbances can be attributed to forces other than the aging process.

While the previous discussion centered on intellectual functioning, what about the elderly person's emotional well-being? Some psychological pathology has been shown in regressive behavior and a tendency of the older adult to become inflexible in his or her personality traits. The senior citizen is often more cautious when taking risks than are younger people, especially when the payoff is predictable and, perhaps, small. But, when the payoff is substantial, there is no age difference in risk taking. Playing the lottery is an example of a substantial payoff, as are sweepstakes mailings that are directed to the elderly.

One detriment of the older person's caution is that it could result in anxiety, which, in turn, could result in delays in making important decisions. For example, when considering whether to see a doctor for a medical complaint, anxiety about hearing a serious diagnosis could cause the person to delay seeking medical help until the disease process becomes severe. Similarly, anxiety-based denial of major signs and symptoms of disease can contribute to the refusal of medical care or to giving an inaccurate or incomplete medical history.

MENTAL HEALTH PROBLEMS

Mental health disorders are not uncommon in the elderly. Many nursing home residents are frequently admitted with a psychiatric diagnosis, usually of organic or physiological nature. A large number of institutionalized older adults have been diagnosed with Alzheimer's disease or other dementia. Patients with dementia will often show abnormal behavior, including paranoia, agitation, insomnia, and depression. Many of these patients will be taking medications to alleviate the clinical signs associated with the dementia. Another condition seen in the elderly, delirium, can also cause abnormal behavior. Similar to dementia, with delerium there is an underlying medical cause for the condition, but when that cause is eliminated, the abnormal behavior abates. For example, fecal impaction or urinary retention can cause delirium. Alleviating the fecal impaction or urinary retention resolves the problem.

A major psychological problem seen in the elderly is depression. With aging, the body's physical state can deteriorate, making independence and self-support increasingly difficult. With the onset of debilitating conditions, depression can worsen, increasing the possibility of suicide.

A contributing factor to depression is the fear of death. The fear of death in the elderly is often no greater than that in the younger adult. However, in the event of a major health concern or severe physical loss, the fear of death can be enhanced. It is usually a terminal illness or underlying depression that triggers an emotional upheaval over facing one's own mortality.

KEY POINT

Depression is common in the elderly and can be caused by a loss of independence, chronic disease, or fear of death.

Coupled with depression, suicide is a major problem among the elderly. Older adults have fewer suicide gestures and more successful suicides than the younger age groups. Prehospital care providers often respond to suicide gestures in younger adults and teens. These gestures are frequently seen as cries for help and may be preceded by warning signs. In the senior population, there may not be any overt warning signs before a suicide attempt. Prehospital care

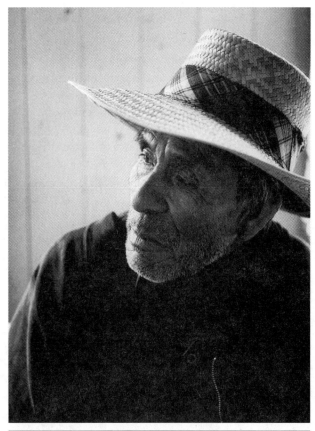

• FIGURE 3-1
Emotional well-being is important. Watch out for the signs of depression in the older adult.

Source: From *Aging,* a magazine of the Administration on Aging, www.oa.dhhs.gov/aoa/magimage/magimage.html.

providers should be aware of the potential for suicide by being familiar with the risk factors. The risk factors for suicide in the elderly population include:

- Over 55 years of age.
- Male.
- Painful illness or disability.
- Lives alone. May have recently lost spouse.
- Loneliness.
- Poverty or economic hardship. May have recently retired or lost job.
- Grief over the loss of a loved one.
- Depression.
- Low self-esteem.
- Drug and/or alcohol abuse.
- Suicide ideation.
- Plan and available means for carrying out a suicide.

As mentioned earlier, depression is a common psychological disorder found in older adults. There are a number of depressive illnesses ranging from a major depressive episode to bipolar disorder. Since the prehospital care provider will not make any differentiation between the variations of depression, this discussion will center on a general description of depression. By definition, depression consists of an altered mood with feelings of despair, sadness, and discouragement.

Signs and symptoms of depression can vary depending on the individual; however, the major indications of depression include:

- Depressed mood or the feeling of being "down" for most, if not all, of the day, nearly every day.
- A significant loss of interest in pleasure. There is no joy in previously enjoyable activities.
- Significant weight loss or gain.
- Insomnia or excessive sleep. Excessive sleep can be an attempt to avoid daily activities or contact with others.
- Restlessness or irritability.
- Fatigue. Simple tasks take a major effort to accomplish.
- Low self-esteem or feelings of worthlessness. A feeling of being a burden to others.
- Indecisiveness or decreased ability to think or concentrate.
- Thoughts of death or suicide ideation.

These clinical signs and symptoms of depression are found in all age groups; however, the older adult differs from the younger depressed patient in several ways. First, the older adult will often complain of general body ailments, whereas the younger adult frequently presents with psychological symptoms. Second, the elderly patient will deny being depressed or having a sad mood. Third, feelings of guilt are not as common in the older adult. Finally, the loss of self-worth is far more predominant in the older patient.

KEY POINT

Be acutely aware of the potential for depression. It negatively impacts patient assessment as the older adult may hide or minimize complaints.

People at risk for depression have several associated risk factors that pre-hospital care providers can recognize when first approaching the patient. The risk factors for depression include:

- Family history of depression. If a family member has been diagnosed with depression, there is an increased risk of depression for the older adult.
- Major events in the patient's life such as recent loss of a loved one, diagnosis of severe or life-threatening disease, chronic pain, or reduced level of function.
- Being isolated from social interaction with others.
- Alcohol use or abuse.
- History of physical abuse or domestic violence.
- Risk factors associated with aging including:
  - Loss of employment or income and loss of respect associated with income or wealth.
  - Change in appearance such as graying of hair and wrinkles.
  - Loss of control over one's life.
  - Loss of control over body functions.
  - Loss of independence or threat of lost independence.

To help evaluate a patient for depression, there are a number of depression-assessment tools available. Although prehospital care providers may not be specifically looking for depression in the elderly patient, the prehospital care provider can ask a few questions that can help screen for depression. A positive

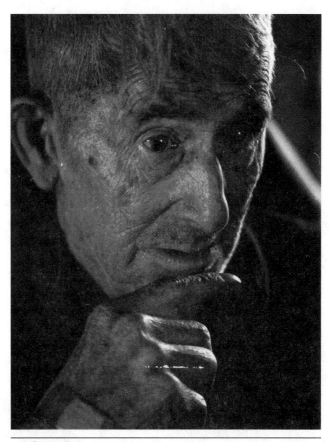

• FIGURE 3-2
Indecisiveness or inability to concentrate could indicate depression.

Source: From *Aging,* a magazine of the Administration on Aging, www.oa.dhhs.gov/aoa/magimage/magimage.html.

finding should be reported to the emergency department physician for continued assessment and, if necessary, referral to a mental health professional. We have provided the Geriatric Depression Scale, a tool that has been used to assess depression in the elderly patient. When on the scene of a medical complaint or while en route to the emergency department, the prehospital care provider can ask some or all of these questions as a screening mechanism for depression.

Geriatric Depression Scale
Choose the Best Answer for How You Felt This Past Week

1. Are you basically satisfied with your life?	Yes	NO
2. Have you discontinued many of your activities and interests?	YES	No
3. Do you feel that your life is empty?	YES	No
4. Do you often get bored?	YES	No
5. Are you hopeful about the future?	Yes	NO
6. Are you bothered by thoughts you cannot get out of your head?	YES	No
7. Are you in good spirits most of the time?	Yes	NO
8. Are you afraid something bad is going to happen to you?	YES	no
9. Do you feel happy most of the time?	yes	NO
10. Do you often feel helpless?	YES	no
11. Do you often get restless or fidgety?	YES	no
12. Do you prefer to stay at home rather than going out?	YES	no
13. Do you frequently worry about the future?	YES	no
14. Do you feel you have more problems with memory than most?	YES	no
15. Do you think it's wonderful to be alive now?	yes	NO
16. Do you often feel pretty downhearted and blue?	YES	no
17. Do you feel worthless the way you are now?	YES	no
18. Do you worry a lot about the past?	YES	no
19. Do you find life very exciting?	yes	NO
20. Is it hard for you to get started on new projects?	YES	no
21. Do you feel full of energy?	yes	NO
22. Do you feel like your situation is hopeless?	YES	no
23. Do you think that most people are better off than you?	YES	no
24. Do you frequently get upset over little things?	YES	no
25. Do you frequently feel like crying?	YES	no
26. Do you have trouble concentrating?	YES	no
27. Do you enjoy getting up in the morning?	yes	NO
28. Do you prefer to avoid social gatherings?	YES	no
29. Is it easy for you to make decisions?	yes	NO
30. Is your mind as clear as it used to be?	yes	NO

Count the number of CAPITALIZED (depression) answers.

Score: _____ (Number of "depressed" answers.)

Norms	
Normal	1–9 (5+/−4)
Mildly depressed	9–21 (15+/−6)
Very depressed	≥18 (23+/−5)

It should be noted that the signs and symptoms of depression can be caused by a variety of illnesses when, in fact, no depression actually exists. For example, Parkinson's disease can result in the outward appearance of depression. It is also interesting to note that some medications can cause the symptoms of depression. A careful history of the patient, including medication use, may give the prehospital care provider some insight into the patient's behavior that can be reported to the emergency department physician. The following table lists medications that may cause the signs and symptoms of depression in the older adult. These drugs are listed by their general use and generic names.

Medications That May Cause Signs of Depression in the Older Adult

Type of Medication	Generic Name	Trade Name
Cardiovascular medications	Clonidine	Catapres
	Digitalis	Lanoxin
	Diuretics	Various
	Hydrazaline	Apresoline
	Lidocaine	Xylocaine
	Methyldopa	Aldomet
	Propranolol	Inderal
	Reserpine	
Pain medications	Morphine	
	Codeine	
	Meperidine	Demerol
	Propoxyphene	Darvon
	Indomethacin	Indocin
Sedatives	Chlordiazepoxide	Librium
	Diazepam	Valium
	Meprobamate	Equanil/Miltown
	Secobartibal	Seconal
	Pentobarbital	Nembutal
Antipsychotics	Haloperidol	Haldol
Steroids	Corticosteroids	
	Estrogen replacements	
Miscellaneous	Cimetidine	Tagamet
	Alcohol	

KEY POINT

Many medications can cause the signs and symptoms of depression. A careful history including prescription and nonprescription drugs is essential.

Many illnesses are associated with depression. By becoming familiar with the diseases associated with depression in the elderly, the prehospital care provider can enhance his or her skills at patient assessment and care. The diseases associated with depression include:

- Acute myocardial infarction
- Anemia
- Arthritis
- Bacterial and viral infections, including pneumonia, tuberculosis, and urinary tract infections
- Bone cancer
- Congestive heart failure
- COPD
- Dehydration
- Dementia
- Diabetes mellitus
- Gastrointestinal cancer
- Hyper- and Hypoglycemia
- Hypoxia
- Lung cancer
- Osteoporosis with fracture
- Stroke
- Transient ischemic attack
- Vitamin deficiencies

KEY POINT

Illness can be associated with depression. A careful history and physical examination of the older patient can suggest associated illnesses.

Along with depression and suicide, another problem associated with the mental health of the elderly is alcohol abuse. Generally, older people consume fewer alcoholic beverages than younger people. However, studies suggest that one to five percent of the over-60 age group may abuse alcohol.

There are three types of elderly drinkers: early-onset drinkers, late-onset drinkers, and intermittent or binge drinkers. The early-onset drinker is one who developed a drinking problem earlier in life. Current beliefs hold that most of the older adults who have a drinking problem belong in this category. The late-onset drinker is one who developed a drinking problem later in life, usually in response to a traumatic event, such as death of a loved one, loss of a job, or other similar event. The late-onset drinker may also drink to dull chronic pain or loneliness. The intermittent or binge drinker only occasionally drinks to excess.

The older adult may turn to alcohol or increase consumption for a variety of reasons. Two of the larger contributing factors to alcohol abuse include a disruption in lifestyle by events such as retirement and decreased social activity. Additionally, loneliness and isolation from others can cause an increase in drinking, as can chronic illness and pain. Some elderly use alcohol to help them sleep or overcome some emotional or physical distress. Unfortunately, what these individuals fail to realize is that excessive use of alcohol can contribute to poor sleep and actually increase depression.

The effects of alcohol are also increased in the older adult. Because of a drop in body water and fat, alcohol is more concentrated in the blood, leading

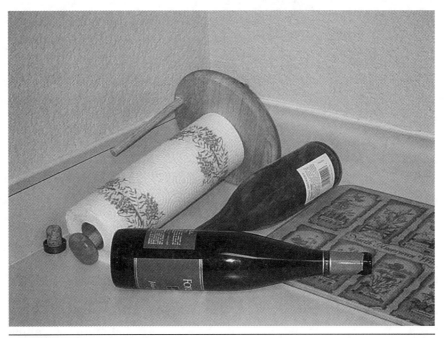

• FIGURE 3-3

Look for evidence of alcohol abuse such as numerous empties strewn about the kitchen, bottles or cans hidden from view, or empty bottles or cans overflowing from the trash container.

KEY POINT

Alcohol abuse is common in older adults. Look for overt and hidden signs of alcohol abuse.

to intoxication at reduced consumption. With decreased blood flow to the liver and reduced liver function, metabolism of alcohol is delayed, prolonging the drug's effects. The effects of alcohol on the brain are also greater. The older adult can become disoriented and lose coordination more readily than a younger adult. Falls and injuries can occur with minimal alcohol consumption. Alcohol can also interact with prescription drugs. CNS depressants, including tranquilizers and pain medications, can have a significantly increased effect in the presence of alcohol. Patients taking antidepressant medications can become even more depressed.

The older adult may hide their alcohol abuse from family members and medical professionals. They often deny any problem with alcohol consumption and destroy any evidence of alcohol use, such as empty bottles or other containers. In one case, EMS was summoned to care for an elderly man whose wife stated he had "vomited blood." Although the prehospital care providers could find no trace of vomit (the woman had cleaned the bathroom), she insisted there was blood in her husband's emesis. On questioning the patient in front of his wife, he adamantly denied alcohol use. He did admit to having a prior problem with drinking and that he was taking Antabuse. Antabuse is a drug given to select alcoholics to "enforce sobriety" since, in the presence of alcohol, it causes a throbbing headache, nausea, and vomiting. While en route to the emergency department and away from his wife, the man admitted that he had been at a friend's home and did have "one beer."

Prehospital care providers should be aware of the potential for alcohol abuse and report any suspicions to the emergency department physician. At times, especially when encountering the binge drinker, the prehospital care provider needs to be prepared to provide acute care that may involve maintaining the airway and providing fluid resuscitation.

EFFECTS OF PSYCHOSOCIAL CHANGES ON PREHOSPITAL CARE

Prehospital care providers will often be called to care for an elderly patient who, along with acute and chronic problems, may also be depressed. Depression or other psychological problems can interfere with prehospital assessment and treatment. To enhance patient evaluation, the prehospital care provider should be aware of how mental disorders can affect the patient's responses to questions.

In some cases, the chief complaint may mask an underlying depression. The patient may call for EMS with a seemingly minor complaint. Prehospital care providers have frequently heard the general complaint of, "I hurt all over," especially in the wee hours of the morning. Patients may also complain of fatigue, restlessness, palpitations, dizziness, or a sense that something is wrong. Altered sensory and pain perception leading to vague complaints are common in the elderly and may lead to frequent calls to 9-1-1. After a complete assessment that fails to find a problem, the patient is reassured. Occasionally, the patient is transported to the emergency department where reassurance is continued, and, since there is no apparent problem, he or she is discharged home. A few days later, the patient again calls for assistance. Repeated calls to 9-1-1 for vague complaints should trigger the suspicion of depression. Report any suspected depression to the emergency department physician.

The patient may also be extremely fearful. One major fear of the elderly is the loss of independence. Many medical conditions such as cancer, stroke, heart disease, and any other debilitating condition could restrict the patient's independent functioning. The fear of loss of independence can be so strong that the patient refuses to acknowledge an illness. Because the patient may not want to face a serious illness, the chief complaint may be trivialized. The patient may refuse assistance or transportation to the hospital.

The patient may also have a strong fear of death. Unless the patient has had some time to emotionally deal with their own mortality, the fear of death could be exaggerated. They may cling onto whatever hope is offered, real or imagined, and seek reassurance from the prehospital care provider whenever possible.

Another mechanism at work is denial. The patient may refuse to accept that anything is wrong. The prehospital care provider must probe for details as to the nature of the complaint. It is important not to become frustrated or to hurry the assessment. In hurrying or rushing the patient evaluation, the prehospital care provider could overlook a critical finding.

Be alert for the signs of depression. In asking about past medical history, check if the patient has been taking any of the well-known antidepressant medi-

> **KEY POINT**
>
> Fear and denial can hinder patient assessment. The older adult may not cooperate during the history and physical examination. Probing for information may be required.

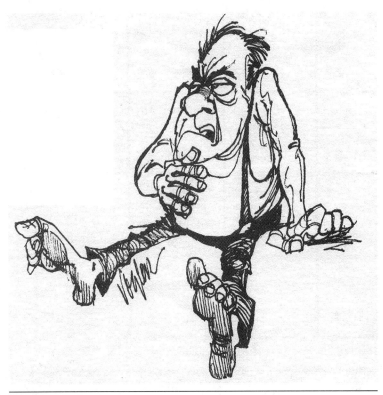

• FIGURE 3-4
The older patient may deny that anything is wrong or may be hostile toward any effort to help.
Source: Courtesy of EES Publications.

cations. Ask specifically if the patient is taking any of the tricyclic antidepressants, the selective serotonin reuptake inhibitors (SSRI), or the monoamine oxidase inhibitors (MAO inhibitors). The following chart contains the names of the more commonly prescribed drugs used to treat depression in the elderly. The medications are listed by brand name.

Common Medications Used to Treat Depression in the Elderly

Type of Medication	Brand Name of Drug
Tricyclic antidepressants	Amitril
	Ascendin
	Aventyl
	Elavil
	Endep
	Norpramin
	Pamelor
	Vivactil
Selective serotonin reuptake inhibitors (SSRI)	Paxil
	Prozac
	Zoloft
Monamine oxidase inhibitors (MOA inhibitors)	Nardil
	Parnate

These medications also have side effects that will be discussed in the chapter on pharmacology in the elderly.

SUMMARY

The prehospital care provider will frequently be called to attend to the geriatric patient. Not only must the prehospital care provider be familiar with the physical changes associated with aging, he or she must also be familiar with the psychological changes and problems seen in the elderly.

Although dementia and delirium are common problems seen in the older adult, many senior citizens are depressed. Depression in the elderly can precede a suicide attempt, and it can interfere with patient assessment and care. Being alert for depression in the senior citizen is an important part of overall patient evaluation and care. The prehospital care provider may be able to recognize the risk factors as well as the signs and symptoms of depression and report depressed patients to the emergency department physician. Early intervention can lead to an improvement of the quality of life for the older adult.

ON THE JOB

You are called to a private home where you find an 80-year-old man sitting on the living room floor. His home is unkempt, with old newspapers, dishes, glasses, and beer cans strewn about. The man is wearing old, dirty jeans and a stained T-shirt. He has not shaved in several days. The man looks at you cautiously and mutters, "What the hell do you want? Nothing wrong here. Just go back when you came from and leave me alone." How would you approach this situation?

4

Patient Assessment

OBJECTIVES

At the end of the chapter, the reader will be able to:

1 List four items in the overall scene survey that could indicate a failure in the patient's ability to provide self-care.

2 List two signs of alcohol abuse that could be seen in the initial scene survey.

3 State 10 things that can enhance communications between the prehospital care provider and the vision-impaired patient.

4 State 14 things that can enhance communications between the prehospital care provider and the hearing-impaired patient.

5 List nine diagnostic signs.

6 Describe the components of the acronym OPQRST when assessing a patient's complaint of pain.

7 Describe the components of the acronym SAMPLE when assessing a patient's current and past medical history.

8 Demonstrate proper questioning and probing for complaints involving specific organ systems.

WORDS TO KNOW

Aortic aneurysm   A sac formed by local dilation of the aorta.

Biot's breathing   Totally irregular breathing pattern.

Cheyne-Stokes breathing   The waxing and waning of breathing followed by a period of apnea.

Cholecystitis   Inflammation of the gall bladder.

Chronic obstructive pulmonary disease (COPD)   A general description for emphysema and chronic bronchitis.

Delirium   A temporary disturbance in consciousness that is accompanied by loss of intellectual functioning and impaired memory.

Dementia   A gradual deterioration in intellectual functioning and memory.

Dorsalis pedis (pedal) pulse   The pulse on the top of the foot.

Heart murmur   A blowing sound heard when listening to the heart tones created by blood flowing through a partially closed heart valve.

Hypothermia   Low core body temperature.

Rales   An abnormal breath sound caused by air moving through fluid. Also called crackles, they are usually heard on inhalation.

Referred pain   Pain felt in an area away from the actual site of tissue damage or injury.

Rhonchi   An abnormal breath sound in the lower airways caused by partial obstruction of the airway. They are typically heard on exhalation and clear upon coughing.

Skin turgor   A reflection of the skin's elasticity and hydration checked by gently pinching then releasing the skin. The skin should return to normal within 3 seconds.

Viscera   A term referring to the internal organs of the body.

Prehospital care providers must perform a thorough assessment on every patient. The assessment is the cornerstone of patient care, because without a patient evaluation, effective care for the person and their condition cannot be provided. Patient evaluation techniques for nearly every patient are well documented in prehospital care provider training programs, therefore, this chapter will focus on patient assessment techniques where the prehospital care provider is evaluating the older adult. The chapter will present information on scene size-up, factors affecting communications, psychological conditions that could affect assessment, and other factors that could influence the evaluation process as they pertain to the older population. It will also discuss the evaluation of a patient's pain and the taking of the patient's current and past medical history.

SCENE SIZE-UP

Upon arrival at the scene of any emergency, prehospital care providers will quickly assess the entire scene for safety and clues to the patient's condition. This includes those times when prehospital care providers are called on to care for an older adult. However, there are some slight differences when sizing-up a situation involving an older adult. In addition to scene safety and hints to the patient's illness or injury, prehospital care providers should look for associated or relevant conditions. For example, in a patient who appears to be having a stroke one should look for evidence of a recent heart attack.

When you arrive at a scene, observe the patient's surroundings. Look around the patient's residence and immediate surroundings to assess the patient's ability for self-care. Mentally ask yourself the following questions:

- Is the area neat and tidy or filthy?
- Is the residence littered with trash?
- Is the kitchen reasonably clean or are dirty dishes piled in the sink?
- Are old newspapers strewn about the home?

Trash or dirty dishes piled in the sink or left throughout the home may indicate difficulty or apathy with regards to self-care. It might also indicate an underlying depression or psychological problem that could interfere with self-care.

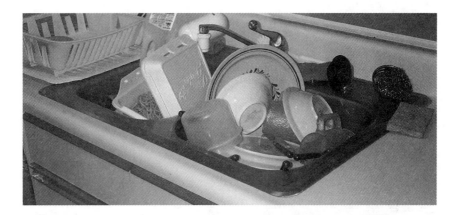

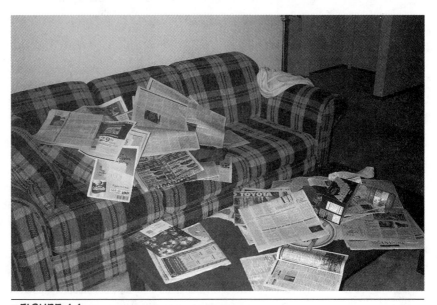

• FIGURE 4-1
Assess patients surroundings for ability for self-care.

When approaching the patient, note the patient's appearance. A disheveled appearance can indicate the patient's inability to care for him- or herself. Keep in mind that not all untidy appearances mean poor self-care. Younger adults can sometimes look unkempt on weekends, when performing yard work or gardening, or when they are not feeling well. Be sure to consider the following:

- Is the hair combed?
- Are the clothes clean or soiled?

In most cases, a pet lifts the spirits of the older adult. Often, the elderly patient treats the pet as a member of the family, in a role similar to that of a child. If, however, the pet has not received proper care, it could reflect on the person's ability to provide self-care.

- Are there animals in the home?
- Have the pets received proper care? Are they well-nourished or emaciated?
- Is there animal excrement inside the home?
- Is there an infestation of fleas?

Alcohol abuse is a serious problem that affects people of all ages. It is prevalent in the elderly and could signal poor self-care, depression, or, perhaps, elder abuse.

- Are there signs of alcohol abuse?
- Are there empty liquor or wine bottles strewn about or in the trash?
- Are there empty beer cans littering the residence or in the trash?

Drugs that are improperly stored or containers that are strewn about the home could indicate poor compliance with the medication regimen. The patient may miss doses or take the drug more often than prescribed, risking an overdose.

- Are medications stored appropriately?
- Are medications in properly labeled containers?

The use of a walking aid such as a cane or walker or the use of a wheelchair does not necessarily mean poor self-care. However, a reduced ability to ambulate could lead to a reduced effort to provide nutrition and hydration.

- Does the patient use walking aids such as a cane or walker?
- Does the patient use a wheelchair?
- Is the patient confined to a wheelchair?

Cold or hot environments can cause hypothermia or heat-related illness. Extremes in temperatures are not needed to induce cold or heat emergencies. Even in appropriate room temperatures a patient's attire could cause excessive heat gain or loss.

- Is the room temperature hot or cold?
- Is the patient dressed appropriately for the temperature?

Elder abuse is a growing problem. The prehospital care provider may be required to report suspicions of abuse to the appropriate authorities. Further, if the prehospital care provider suspects abuse, the provider might have to modify the patient evaluation to reduce the patient's risk of later reprisal.

- Are there indications of physical abuse?
- Are there indications of emotional abuse?
- Are there indications of neglect?

COMMUNICATING WITH THE PATIENT

After the initial assessment of the overall scene and first contact with the patient, prehospital care providers should consider the effects of aging as they relate to the provider's ability to communicate with the patient. Older patients may have diminished sight, hearing, and mental status, which could make patient assessment more difficult. It is important to remember that not all older adults are sight or hearing impaired. It is not necessary to talk loudly to all older patients. Additionally, if a person has low vision or diminished hearing, it is not safe to assume any other sense is affected. In essence, if a patient is blind, do not assume the patient is deaf!

A patient with diminished sight may be afraid of everything that is happening. Rapid movements by EMS personnel can be intimidating. The following list provides some helpful hints for the prehospital care provider dealing with a patient who has low vision or is blind.

- When entering the patient's location, announce who you are and why you are there. Also introduce other members of the EMS crew.
- If there are several people arriving on the scene at the same time, keep movements slow and deliberate, discussing them with the patient.
- Ask if the patient wears glasses and, if so, make sure the patient is wearing them.
- Do not assume that a blind or sight-impaired patient is deaf. There is no need to use a loud voice with a sight-impaired patient.
- Turn down extraneous noise. Lower the volume on dispatch and medical control radios as well as the cardiac monitor. If a stereo is playing, turn it off. Have one person ask questions and coordinate patient care.
- Talk directly to the patient. Unless an interpreter is needed, do not use an intermediary. For example, if the patient is able to respond, do not ask the patient's spouse about the patient's condition (e.g., "Mrs. Jones, how is your husband feeling today?").
- Position yourself where the patient can see you. Many sight-impaired patients have some visual function. If the patient is totally blind, let the person know your location. If you are going to move, let the patient know beforehand (e.g., "Mr. Smith, I am going to your left side."), then change locations.
- Avoid glare or extremely bright lights. Glare is caused by light reflecting from shiny surfaces and can impair vision in the older person. Although bright light can interfere with the patient's ability to see, it is not necessary to turn the lights off.

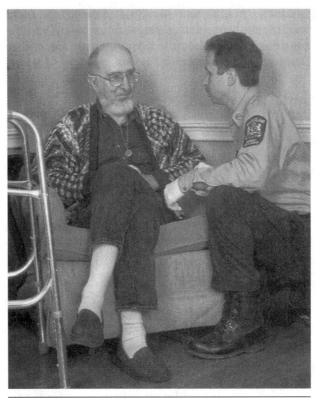

• FIGURE 4-2
Assess patient care at the patient's eye level and look directly at the patient.
Source: Courtesy Brady *Emergency Care*, 8th ed., p. 265.

- Unless absolutely necessary, avoid standing behind the patient. Kneel or sit beside or in front of the patient.
- If leaving the patient's immediate area, for example, to check for medications in the bathroom, let the patient know. Inform the patient when you return to their side.
- Do not move furniture without telling the patient. When the patient returns home, they may have difficulties with rearranged furniture.

KEY POINT

Communicate directly with a patient who has visual impairment. Avoid extraneous noise as the visually impaired person may rely heavily on hearing.

Hearing loss can also affect communications and hamper patient assessment. Hearing loss occurs due to natural deterioration with age or because of damage from occupational conditions. Patients may also have a condition known as tinnitus, or ringing in the ears, which hinders hearing. With gradual hearing loss, many people will begin to read lips to enhance their remaining hearing. Many older adults use hearing devices fitted inside the ear canal or around the outside of the ear. If the patient has a hearing loss, the following tips will help the prehospital care provider communicate more effectively with the patient.

- High frequencies are the first to go. The patient may be better able to hear the male voice.
- Ask if the patient uses a hearing aid. If so, make sure the patient is wearing and using it.
- Be on the same level as the hearing-impaired patient and face them directly. Look at the patient when you are talking.
- Make sure that any light is shining on the speaker's face, not into the eyes of the patient.
- Reduce background noise from the television or radio, dispatch radio, and cardiac monitor.
- Select one person to talk with the patient. Several people asking questions at once will confuse and irritate the patient.
- Never talk to the person from another room or from behind. Be sure to get the patient's attention before speaking. Calling the person by name helps get the person's attention.
- Avoid talking quickly or using long, complex sentences. Pause between sentences or phrases.
- Remember that when ill or tired, hearing-impaired people do not hear and understand as well.
- If a patient has trouble understanding something, try saying it in a different way using different words rather than repeating the same words.
- Speak as clearly and accurately as possible. Do not shout or "overmouth" words. Shouting or exaggerated mouth movement distorts the words, making them harder for the hearing-impaired person to understand. Do not drop your voice or lower your tone at the end of a sentence.
- Although this should go without mentioning, do not eat, chew gum or candy, or smoke while talking. This interferes with mouth movements and can confuse the patient who reads lips.
- Keep your hands away from your face. Do not put pens into your mouth or cover your mouth with your hands or fingers while you are speaking.
- When giving specific information, have the patient repeat the information back to you to ensure that it has been understood.
- When changing the topic, be sure to tell the patient. For example, say "We are talking about __ now."
- If necessary, use a pen and paper to write questions.

KEY POINT

A large number of older adults are hearing impaired. Speak clearly and directly to the patient without exaggerating words or mouth movements. If necessary, use written notes.

PATIENTS WITH DIMINISHED MENTAL STATUS

Not only will impaired hearing or vision affect assessments, patients with diminished mental status pose a special problem for the prehospital care provider. Responses to questions may be delayed while a patient processes the information. This delay in response could be due to a medical condition, such as a stroke, that has affected the patient's mental status. It could also be due to medications

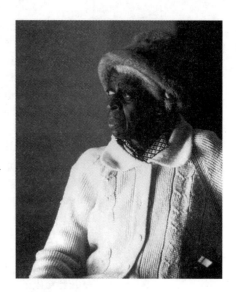

• FIGURE 4-3
Assessing a patient with a diminished mental state can be a challenge.

Source: From *Aging,* a magazine of the Administration on Aging, www.aoa.dhhs.gov/aoa/magimage/magimage.html.

that slow the patient's response. It may be necessary to wait a few moments for the older adult to process the question and formulate an answer. Prehospital care providers should ask questions slowly and precisely and then allow the older patient time to respond. Failure to respond quickly is not always abnormal.

Older patients may not appropriately respond to questions. For example, if asked, "How are you feeling today?" the patient may reply with, "My kitty is playing outside and may be hungry." Should this occur, ascertaining appropriate medical information could be difficult at best. It might be necessary to rely upon the patient's family or caregiver to shed light on the patient's past and present medical history. It is important to not become frustrated. For more information on dealing with patients with dementia and delirium, see Chapter 5.

As was discussed in Chapter 3, older adults may also suffer from depression. Depressed patients may trivialize complaints, not wanting to be a "bother" for EMS personnel. The prehospital care provider may have to probe for significant problems as the patient may not be willing to volunteer relevant information. The patient may also have thoughts of suicide. If the patient suggests suicide as an option, saying "I think I will end it all so my kids won't have to put up with me," the prehospital care provider should take the comment seriously and report it to the emergency department physician. It is also important to note that the call for assistance may have resulted from a suicide gesture such as an overdose of medication.

Finally, as with younger patients, the older adult may deny any medical emergency. Remember, the senior may think that medical problems will cause a loss of independence or function, so admitting that there is an illness could be associated with giving up independence. The patient may not want to give all the information necessary to assess the condition or may minimize any symptoms such as pain. The older adult may also refuse treatment and transportation to the hospital. The prehospital care provider may have to solicit help from family, friends, or the patient's personal physician to convince the patient to go to the hospital.

OTHER FACTORS IN ASSESSMENT

The prehospital care provider should consider other factors that could impact the efficiency of the patient evaluation. The patient may become fatigued easily. Although the aging process can affect a patient's stamina, medical conditions such as pneumonia can cause the patient to become more easily fatigued.

If the patient shows signs of slowing, such as in their response to questions, ask if they are getting tired. If the patient is tired, try a different approach, wait patiently for the patient's responses, or change procedures altogether.

It may be necessary to differentiate the acute emergency from a chronic condition, as well as to identify multiple systems problems. At times, the chronic condition will be the root of the acute problem. For example, if the patient has a history of COPD, is it related to the patient's current chest discomfort? For example, is mental confusion in a known diabetic patient caused by hypoglycemia? Finally, patients may attribute some problems to "just getting older."

Because some older adults hoard medications, it might be necessary to separate currently used drugs from those the patient is "storing" for future use. Look at expiration dates, count the number of pills remaining in the bottle, and, if necessary, ask the patient if a medication is current.

THE DIAGNOSTIC SIGNS

Once the scene has been evaluated and communications with the patient established, the prehospital care provider will begin a hands-on patient assessment that includes the diagnostic signs as well as a head-to-toe survey of the body. The diagnostic signs are important, as they will provide information on the patient's mental state, circulatory status, and clues as to the cause of the patient's distress.

Level of Consciousness

The patient's level of consciousness will give clues as to his or her mental state and the circulatory status of the brain. Many prehospital care providers will use the mnemonic *AVPU* to assess level of consciousness. The AVPU mnemonic stands for the following:

A Alert and oriented to person, place, time, and situation
V Alert and responsive to verbal stimulation
P Alert and responsive to painful (physical) stimulation
U Unconscious

In lieu of the AVPU mnemonic, the prehospital care provider could use the Glasgow Coma Scale to assess level of responsiveness. However, some older patients may not respond as younger adults do. For example, the patient with dementia may not be oriented to person, place, time, and situation. Although the response may be abnormal for the younger adult, it could be perfectly acceptable in the patient with Alzheimer's disease. A patient with delirium may also fail to respond appropriately to questions pertaining to person, place, time, and situation. In either case, ask family members or caregivers about the normal mental status of the patient. Always remember to consider underlying chronic illnesses that could affect mental status.

Breathing

Assess the patient's breathing for rate, depth, and rhythm. While the normal breathing rates for adults range from 12 to 20 breaths per minute, older adults, especially those with COPD, can have lower- or higher-than-normal ventilatory rates. For example, a patient with chronic bronchitis may take 8 to 10 breaths per minute. In contrast, a patient with emphysema may breathe faster than normal. Prehospital care providers should not rely solely on ventilatory rate to determine adequacy of ventilation.

Like the rate, the depth of breathing may vary in the older adult. Because of a decreased vital capacity, the older adult may take shallow breaths instead of full, deep breaths. As with breathing rate, the prehospital care provider should assess other factors and not determine ventilatory effectiveness based solely upon depth of breathing.

The ventilatory rhythm should be regular. Abnormal rhythms such as Cheyne-Stokes or Biot's breathing indicates potential CNS damage or disease and requires further assessment and intervention.

Assessment of breath sounds is equally important in both younger and older adults. With aging and a reduction in vital capacity, breath sounds may be more difficult to hear. Adventitious sounds such as rales, rhonchi, and wheezes could be normal for the patient depending on their underlying condition. For example, a patient with COPD may have fine rales or crackles that could be confused with pneumonia or the early stages of pulmonary edema. Abnormal breath sounds should stimulate questions pertaining to the patient's past medical history as well as to underlying chronic conditions.

Pulse

The patient's heart rate, pulse strength or force, and heart rhythm should be checked. The normal heart rate ranges from 60 to 100 beats per minute in the average-aged adult. In the older adult, a slower heart rate may be normal. The regularity of the heartbeat should also be noted. A regular rhythm, although normal, is not always typical in the older adult. A senior citizen can have premature beats that are normal for him or her. When finding an irregular pulse, ask the patient if they have ever been told of an irregular heartbeat. Monitor the patient's ECG. An occasional premature atrial or ventricular contraction is normal. However, be sure to note any abnormal cardiac rhythms.

When possible, take the patient's pulse when the patient is supine, then again when the patient is sitting. Significant increases in heart rate equal to or greater than 15–20 beats per minute from the supine to a sitting position could indicate orthostatic hypotension. This should be noted on the patient care report as well as reported to the emergency department physician.

Keep in mind that the older patient's response to shock is slower. As discussed in Chapter 3, the heart rate change of an older adult in response to hypotension may be half that of the younger adult. Older patients, especially those

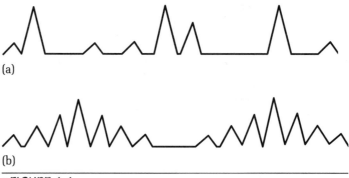

(a)

(b)

• FIGURE 4-4
(a) Biot's Breathing—Totally irregular breathing pattern.
(b) Cheyne-Stoke's Breathing—Waxing and waning of breathing with periods of apnea.

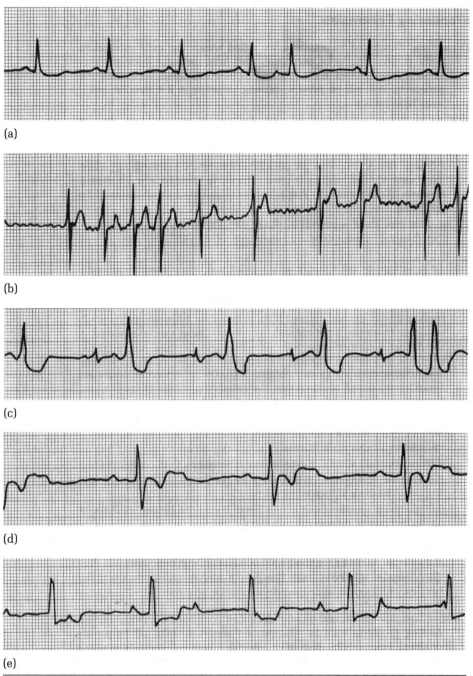

(a)

(b)

(c)

(d)

(e)

• FIGURE 4-5

Abnormal cardiac rhythms (a) premature atrial contraction (b) atrial fibrillation (c) premature ventricular contractions (d) second degree AV block-Type II (e) third degree AV block.

Source: Courtesy Brady *Paramedic Emergency Care*, pp. 640–662.

KEY POINT

An irregular heart rhythm in the older patient could be normal. Ask the patient if the doctor has told them of an irregular heartbeat. Check the patient's ECG, if necessary.

with polypharmacy, can have a depressed response to a drop in blood pressure. Consider patients on beta blocker drugs for hypertension; a drop in blood pressure from shock may be met with little or no increase in heart rate. Thus, an older adult who is hypotensive may have a normal heart rate.

Peripheral pulses may be difficult to find. Conditions such as atherosclerosis and arteriosclerosis may make palpation of a dorsalis pedis (pedal) pulse nearly impossible. Long-term diabetics may have such poor circulation to the feet that a pedal pulse may only be found by Doppler assessment—a tool that EMS crews rarely carry. If a peripheral pulse cannot be located, it is not safe to assume the pulse does not exist. The prehospital care provider must rely on other findings, such as color and temperature, to more completely assess distal circulation.

Listening to the patient's heart sounds is also beneficial. Blood rushing up against closed valves causes the normal heart tones. When these valves are damaged or diseased, heart murmurs can develop. A blowing sound heard when the heart contracts indicates a heart murmur. In some older adults, a murmur is normal, but it can be a contributing factor to a number of conditions, such as congestive heart failure. As with an irregular heart rhythm, ask the patient if they have been told about any heart murmur.

Blood Pressure

Assess the patient's blood pressure to determine both systolic and diastolic pressures. The normal blood pressure for average-aged adults is based on the following calculation:

	Men	**Women**
Systolic	Age +100	Age +90
Diastolic	80–90	70–80

With aging, the blood pressure increases to well above 140/90. As will be discussed in the chapter on medical emergencies, an elevation in the systolic blood pressure may be a more significant prognosticator of cardiovascular disease than the diastolic blood pressure. If a patient has an elevated blood pressure, the prehospital care provider should ask about the patient's normal blood pressure. Also, prehospital care providers should remember that, in an older adult, a blood pressure of 110/70 could be hypotensive.

KEY POINT

An older patient with what appears to be a normal blood pressure could be in shock. Ask if the patient knows their normal blood pressure.

When possible, take the patient's blood pressure when the patient is supine, then again when the patient is sitting. Significant decreases in blood pressure ($\leq$20/10 mm Hg) from a supine to a sitting position could indicate orthostatic hypotension and should be noted on the patient care report as well as reported to the emergency department physician.

Skin Color, Condition, and Temperature

Assessment of the skin color, condition, and temperature can give the prehospital care provider an indication of peripheral blood flow. However, in the older adult, what might be considered abnormal in the younger person might be a normal finding. Skin color is normally pink with some other coloration depending on ambient temperature. However, in the senior citizen, pale skin may be the norm. Decreased circulation to the skin, as well as reduced sun exposure, keeps the skin somewhat pale.

Skin condition involves the moisture in and on the skin. Skin turgor, as mentioned in Chapter 3, is altered in the older adult. With age, the skin's elasticity decreases as collagen support deteriorates. Tenting the skin on the back of the hand of an older adult will result in prolonged tenting, even when the patient is normally hydrated. To check for skin turgor in the older patient, gently pinch the skin on the patient's cheek, forehead, chest, or abdomen.

Moisture on the skin depends on the functioning of the patient's sweat glands. With age, the number of working sweat glands decreases. A patient's skin may be drier than expected in times of exposure to warm temperatures. If the skin does not sweat, the ability of the senior citizen to reduce body heat through evaporation decreases, and the person is at an increased risk for heat stroke.

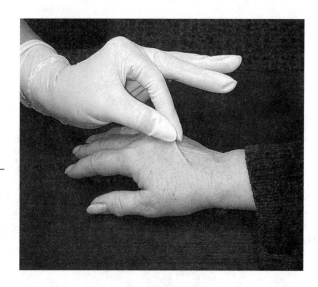

• FIGURE 4-6
Tenting the skin on the back of the hand to assess turgor is fine in the younger adult. In the older adult, loss of elasticity may give a false positive result.

Patients who might normally be profusely diaphoretic when experiencing a stroke, acute myocardial infarction, or shock may only have slightly moist skin.

Skin temperature, as with skin color, frequently depends on the amount of blood flow to the skin. When blood flow to the skin is normal, the skin is warm. When blood flow has been reduced, the skin is cool to the touch. In the older adult with decreased circulation to the skin, the prehospital care provider may find skin temperature cooler than expected. The decrease in circulation to the skin also contributes to a higher risk of heat stroke among older adults.

Pupils

Checking the pupil response to light is a standard procedure for all prehospital care providers. In the older adult, the pupil response will be different than in the younger adult. As people age, the pupils become smaller and allow less light to pass through. They also react more slowly to changes in light.

> **KEY POINT**
>
> Pupil response to light slows with age. A slow-to-react pupil may be normal in the older adult.

Reaction to Pain

Another diagnostic sign is reaction to pain or merely the presence of pain. Pain is defined as agony, distress, or suffering and is caused by the stimulation of specialized sensory nerves. Pain is protective in nature as it serves as a warning that tissues or body structures are being damaged. Before discussing pain in the older patient, let us first consider a few misunderstandings, or myths, about pain.

Myth: Patients in pain always have a cause for the pain.

Fact: Patients in pain may not have any demonstrable cause for the pain. For example, a patient with a brain tumor has a demonstrable cause for pain, yet a patient with a tension headache has nothing that can be shown as a cause of the pain.

Myth: A person with a low tolerance for pain is often one who has little self-control.

Fact: Tolerance for pain is considered the amount of pain a patient will endure before seeking relief. There are physical reactions to the pain, which are complicated by emotional or psychological factors. Patients who are preoccupied with other tasks during the day may not be distracted by the pain or seek help until the tasks are removed. Once the patient has nothing to distract them from the pain, they often seek relief. Consider the patient who doesn't call 9-1-1 until late at night even though they have been in pain for most of the day. After going to bed and not having something to take their mind off of the discomfort, the endurance factor is reduced.

Myth: The perception of pain decreases as a person gets older.

Fact: Unless a person's nervous system is impaired due to illness such as a stroke or injury or neuropathy, the perception of pain remains the same for all ages. In essence, if it hurts at age 40, it will still hurt the same at age 80. Some patients may not be able to effectively communicate the nature and intensity of the pain effectively due to a stroke or other CNS problem, but the pain is still present.

Myth: Narcotic medications should not be administered to the older patient.

Fact: Although older adults may not be able to biotransform (see chapter on pharmacology) the medication as quickly and effectively as younger adults, age is not a contraindication to the use of narcotic pain medication. Because of the age-related changes in metabolism, give seniors lower doses and titrate to effect.

There are three major types or descriptions of pain: pricking pain, burning pain, and aching pain. Although other terms have been used to describe pain, such as throbbing, cramping, and electric, the three major types can be used to allow the patient to more precisely describe their discomfort. Pricking pain is best described as the pain associated with pricking the skin with a needle or cutting the skin with a knife. It can be sharp and severe. Burning pain is the sensation that occurs when the skin is, as the name implies, burned. It can be a very severe pain. Aching pain is typically felt deep inside the body. It can vary in intensity and, if diffuse, can be severe.

KEY POINT

Asking about the quality of the pain can give insight to the location of the pain. Pricking and burning pain is more superficial, whereas aching pain tends to originate from an organ.

In addition to the three types of pain, there is also a difference between pain at the surface of the body (skin) and that at the organs (viscera). Visceral pain, or pain in the organs of the body, is caused by stimulation of the pain sensors in those organs. The organs have sensors only for the sensation of pain, and these sensors are diffuse. Localized injury to an organ may actually cause little pain. For example, a stab wound to the abdomen may produce little pain from an injured intestine. (The pricking pain from the cut skin and muscle can be intense.) However, widespread stimulation of the pain sensors in the organs can produce extreme pain in the patient.

Organ pain has several causes. The first is ischemia, or loss of blood flow. When blood flow to an organ or area of an organ is interrupted, the metabolic by-products produced by ischemic tissues stimulate the pain sensors. Pain from a myocardial infarction is a good example of ischemic visceral pain.

Organ pain can also be caused by chemical irritation. For example, if a patient has an ulcer that perforates and leaks gastric contents into the abdomen, chemical irritation throughout the abdomen occurs. The gastric acids attempt to "digest" large areas of the peritoneum, causing the severe pain associated with peritonitis.

If a hollow organ such as the intestine goes into a spasm, that spasm causes cramping visceral pain. The exact mechanism of this pain is not absolutely clear, as the pain could be a mechanical stimulation of the pain sensors or it could be the result of the spasm reducing the blood flow (ischemia) to the affected tissue.

Organ pain can also be the result of distention of a hollow organ. If the tissues of the hollow organ become stretched and distended, pain results. Pain can also result from the collapse of blood vessels in the distended organ.

KEY POINT

Consider the possible source of the organ pain. Ischemia, chemical irritation, and spasms can cause organ pain.

Patients may often complain of pain in an area of the body that is not associated with the organ that may be damaged or injured. This phenomenon is known as referred pain or radiation of pain. The reason for this is that the pain sensations are transmitted to the spinal cord by way of some of the same nerve cells that transmit pain sensations from the skin. Because the nerve pathways are the same, the brain may have trouble identifying the exact source of the pain. The person then feels pain at the level of the skin. It is important to note the presence of referred pain, because some patients may have no other pain sensations. For example, a diabetic patient with an acute myocardial infarction may not have any chest discomfort, yet feel pain in their lower jaw or left arm. The following diagram illustrates some of the areas associated with referred pain.

The perception of pain can be affected by a number of factors, including neuropathies or central nervous system impairment. As mentioned in our discussion of the myths of pain, if the patient's central nervous system is functioning normally, the patient will feel pain normally. If there has been significant

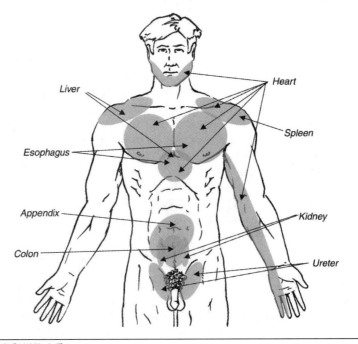

• FIGURE 4-7

Sites of pain based upon diseased or injured organs.

Source: Courtesy Brady *MedEMT*, p. 137.

damage to the central nervous system, the sensation of pain may be altered. Another alteration of pain sensation occurs if the patient has neuropathies such as diabetic neuropathy. In such cases, the perception of pain may be diminished or absent. For example, patients with neuropathies may not experience chest pain from injuries or illness.

KEY POINT

Patients with neuropathy such as diabetic neuropathy may not experience pain. A "silent" heart attack is more common in diabetic patients.

In assessing a patient's pain, many prehospital care providers use one of two acronyms—OPQRST or PAIN. When using either acronym, the prehospital care provider will ask questions associated with the characteristics of the discomfort. The following list explains the OPQRST acronym.

O Onset   When did the pain begin? What were you doing when the pain started?

P Provoke   Was there anything that caused the pain to begin? For example, if the patient has chest pain, is the pain associated with physical exertion? Is there anything that makes the pain better or worse?

Q Quality   What does the pain feel like? Is the pain sharp or stabbing, a burning sensation, or achy? Keep in mind that medications, CNS damage, and neuropathies may alter the sensations.

R Radiation   Does the pain radiate to another area? Is there any referred pain?

S Severity   Using a scale of 1 to 10 with 10 the most severe, how severe is the pain? Again, CNS injury, some drugs, and neuropathies may alter the perception of pain.

T Time   How long has the pain been present?

The acronym PAIN also represents questions the prehospital care provider can ask about the nature, type, and quality of the discomfort.

P Period of the Pain   What started the pain and how long has the pain persisted?

A Area   Where does it hurt most? Is there any referred or radiated pain? Does the pain travel to another part of the body?

I Intensity   How severe is the pain? (Use a rating scale as described in the previous list.) How does the pain feel—sharp, stabbing, burning, achy? Does the pain remain the same or does it change? As mentioned earlier, CNS injury or illness can alter perception of the intensity of pain.

N Nullify   Does anything make the pain better or worse? Have you taken anything for the pain? Did it help?

The diagnostic signs are only a component of a thorough patient assessment. The prehospital care provider will also need to ask about the patient's chief complaint as well as their current and past medical history. A frequently used acronym that serves as a reminder of the questions to ask is SAMPLE.

S Symptoms   Symptoms are subjective findings that the patient reveals such as pain or shortness of breath. Symptoms are things that cannot be seen or felt by the prehospital care provider. Open-ended questions such as "How are you feeling?" invite the patient to respond with a description of their complaint. With elderly patients, they often have a multitude of problems that can precipitate a general answer of "Not so good" or "I hurt all over." The prehospital care provider may have to narrow the question to very specific complaints such as "Are you nauseated?" or "Have you thrown up?" Older adults may minimize complaints, thinking that their aches and pains are part of growing older. They may also fear the loss of independence and disability. Prehospital care providers will have to probe for information and ask specific questions about the various organs. See the following section concerning assessment of the various organ systems. *S* can also refer to "signs," something, such as cyanosis, that is seen during the assessment.

A Allergies   Allergies or allergic reactions to medications are important to note and record on the patient care report. Some people consider adverse reactions to medications as allergies. For example, a patient may state that they are allergic to aspirin because it causes heartburn. Any adverse reactions to prescriptions, over-the-counter drugs, and herbal remedies should be noted and reported.

M Medications   Gathering information on medication can be a lengthy process when evaluating the older patient. With the number of prescription drugs that a senior takes, the patient might not remember all of the medications the doctor has prescribed. It might be helpful to look in the medicine or kitchen cabinets for currently used medications. The prehospital care provider may also want to inquire if the patient knows why they are taking a particular drug. This information can be used as a basis to inquire about the patient's past medical history.

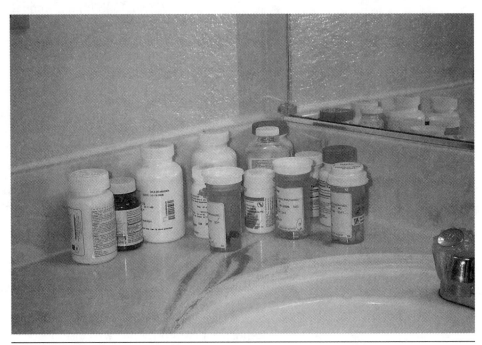

• FIGURE 4-8
Look in the bathroom or other places for medications.

P Previous Illness   Are you under a doctor's care for any medical condition? Have you been treated for any medical problem in the past year? Have you had any recent surgeries or operations? The prehospital care provider may have to probe to get appropriate details pertaining to past medical history; especially as it pertains to the current illness.

L Last Meal or Oral Intake   When was the last time you ate or had anything to drink? What did you eat or drink? Patients may not be eating properly and could be malnourished. Patients with diabetes who are taking their medications but not eating could be at risk for hypoglycemia. If the patient has not been eating properly, the prehospital care provider may want to ask why. The patient who is depressed may not want or feel the need to eat. Further, some medications may inhibit the appetite or cause the patient to have a strange taste in their mouth. In addition to asking when the patient last ate, the prehospital care provider should ask when the patient last had a bowel movement or urinated. Fecal and urinary retention can cause confusion or delirium in the older adult.

E Events Prior to the Incident   What exactly happened before the incident? What were you doing just prior to the problem? Have you done anything to feel better? Does anything make it worse?

PROBING FOR SYMPTOMS

Because older adults tend to underreport medical problems for a variety of reasons, prehospital care providers need to investigate an elderly patient's vague complaints by asking specific questions. An easy and orderly way to probe for information is to ask about specific organ systems. The following are some questions that can be asked when reviewing each organ system.

Respiratory system

Have you had trouble breathing more often than usual?

Do you cough more at night?

Do you have trouble breathing when laying flat that goes away when you sit up?

Do you have a cough that has lasted a long time or has been persistent?

Have you coughed up any mucous or blood?

Cardiovascular system

Have you noticed any unusual swelling in your ankles and feet?

Has your abdomen felt full or bloated recently?

Do you have chest pain or discomfort that goes away?

Does your angina seem to be coming on more often?

Have you noticed some funny feelings or heartbeats in your chest?

Have you noticed any irregular heartbeats?

Have you been getting dizzy or lightheaded?

Have you suddenly fainted recently?

Central Nervous system

Have you noticed any visual disturbances such as blurred vision that goes away?

Have you noticed any visual disturbances that seem to be getting worse?

Have you been walking OK or have you been falling lately?
Have you noticed any unusual weakness in your arms or legs?
Have you felt any strange sensations in your arms or legs?

Gastrointestinal system

Have you been eating normally?
When was the last time you had anything to eat?
Have you had any trouble swallowing?
Have you had any abdominal pain or cramps?
Have you noticed any change in your bowel such as constipation or diarrhea?
Have you noticed any blood when you have a bowel movement?

Genitourinary system

Have you noticed any change in the frequency that you have to urinate?
Have you noticed any bleeding when you urinate?
Have you noticed any vaginal bleeding?

Musculoskeletal system

Do you have any pain in your arms or hands?
Do you have any pain in your legs, ankles, or feet?

Inquiring about signs and symptoms is important, but so is a head-to-toe assessment. While asking about various signs and symptoms, the prehospital care provider can perform a hands-on evaluation of the patient and look for injuries or signs of illness. The procedures for a head-to-toe assessment in the geriatric patient are the same as those for younger patients.

HELPFUL SIGNS

Looking for particular signs or hints to a specific condition sometimes facilitates patient evaluation. Some of these signs can increase the prehospital care provider's index of suspicion to a potentially life-threatening condition. The following are a few signs that indicate an acute, emergent condition.

Aortic aneurysm

When listening to the chest, a double heartbeat is heard. (Robertson's sign)
The patient's head shows a rhythmic jerking motion. (Musset's sign)
A friction sound is heard over the sternum when the patient raises then drops his or her arms. (Perez's sign)
A rhythmic murmur is heard when a stethoscope is applied to the patient's lips. (Sansom's sign)

Cardiac problems

A heart attack may be indicated if the patient holds a clenched fist over the lower sternum. (Levine's sign)
The pectoral muscle over the heart appears to quiver. This could indicate approaching death due to cardiac disease. (Robertson's sign)

Cholecystitis

Press the fingers on the abdomen at the right intercostal margin and have the patient take a deep breath. While taking a deep breath, the patient will abruptly stop inhaling. (Murphy's sign)

Elevated intracranial pressure

Increased blood pressure, bradycardia, and abnormal breathing can indicate rising intracranial pressure. (Cushing's triad)

Ruptured spleen

Severe pain in the left shoulder when no obvious injury is noted indicates a ruptured spleen. (Kehr's sign)

Pain

When pressure is applied to a painful area, the heart rate increases. (Mannkopf's sign)
The pupils will dilate with pressure over a painful area.

Pericardial tamponade

Three findings associated with pericardial tamponade are hypotension, jugular venous distention, and muffled heart tones. (Beck's triad)

SUMMARY

Many years ago, Sir William Osler, a physician and professor of medicine in the United States and Canada, said, "Listen to the patient. He will give you the diagnosis." This statement is true regardless of the age of the patient. By listening to the patient, the prehospital care provider will learn a wealth of information that identifies the nature of the patient's problem. Patient assessment involves talking with the patient and listening to their chief complaint, as well as eliciting a careful history of present and past illnesses.

This chapter has highlighted patient assessment techniques to be considered when evaluating the older adult. It has included information on scene survey as well as techniques for effectively communicating with the hearing- or vision-impaired patient. This chapter also discussed the diagnostic signs and two acronyms for assessing the patient's pain. Finally, an acronym was presented as a guide to evaluating the patient's current and past medical history. Once the patient has been evaluated, the prehospital care provider can determine the necessary emergency care for the ill or injured older adult.

ON THE JOB

You respond to a call for help, and, upon arriving at the 70-year-old man's home, you note the apartment is cluttered with trash, dirty dishes, and cat feces. The smell of cat excrement is nearly overwhelming. Empty wine and liquor bottles are on the dining room and coffee tables amidst stacks of old, unread newspapers. What are some key aspects regarding the man's health that you would ask about or assess?

5

Alzheimer's Dementia and Delirium

OBJECTIVES

At the end of the chapter, the reader will be able to:

1 Define dementia.
2 List six of the nine diagnostic criteria for dementia.
3 Define the terms apraxia, aphasia, and agnosia.
4 List the four categories of dementia.
5 List at least six diagnostic criteria of Alzheimer's disease.
6 List the 10 questions asked on the Short Portable Mental Status Questionnaire.
7 Describe the clinical presentation in each of the four stages of Alzheimer's disease.
8 Differentiate between Alzheimer's disease and multi-infarct dementia.
9 List the terms associated with the acronym DEMENTIA.
10 Differentiate between delirium and dementia.
11 List at least six possible causes of reversible dementia.
12 Define benign senescent forgetfulness.
13 Explain why it may be important to speak slowly to a patient with Alzheimer's disease.
14 Describe three steps in handling aggressive or assaultive behavior displayed by a patient with Alzheimer's disease.
15 Explain the Rule of 5s as it pertains to communicating with a patient with Alzheimer's disease.
16 List two currently accepted drug therapies for Alzheimer's disease.

WORDS TO KNOW

Acetylcholine   An important chemical of the autonomic nervous system.

Agnosia   Inability to recognize familiar people or objects.

Antioxidant   A chemical that prevents or alleviates excessive oxygenation or the creation of free oxygen radicals inside the body—a process that has been attributed to tissue damage.

Aphasia   Inability to communicate effectively by speaking, writing, or sign communications.

Apraxia   Inability to carry out simple motor functions.

Benign senescent forgetfulness   Simple forgetfulness.

Cholinesterase   An enzyme that breaks down acetylcholine and prevents the chemical from acting on nerve cells.

Cognitive functions   Function that involve knowing, perceiving, or remembering.

Delusions   A false belief that is maintained despite contradictory evidence.

Dementia   Loss of cognitive functions over a period of time.

Fecal impaction   Accumulation of hardened feces in the rectum.

Ginko biloba   An over-the-counter herbal remedy that has been shown to improve memory and may assist victims of Alzheimer's disease.

Hallucinations   A sensory perception (sight, sound, smell, taste, touch) that has no basis in external stimulation.

Hemiparesis   Weakness on one side of the body.

Hemiplegia   Paralysis on one side of the body.

Huntington's chorea   Hereditary disease characterized by jerking movements, speech disturbances, and mental deterioration.

Hypercapnia   Excessive carbon dioxide levels in the arterial blood.

Hypoxia   Abnormally low oxygen levels in the arterial blood.

Multi-infarct dementia   Dementia caused by multiple strokes or TIAs.

Parkinson's disease   Progressive disease characterized by deterioration of certain areas of the brain.

Transient ischemic attack (*TIA*)   Temporary block in the blood flow to an area of the brain. Mimics a stroke, but resolves within minutes.

Urosepsis   System-wide septic poisoning caused by retaining or absorbing urinary substances.

Over the past several years, the media have paid increasing attention to a severe and progressive condition that has no cure. This disease has afflicted millions of people, including a past president of the United States. This disease robs a person of their memory and ultimately ends in death. This is not an infectious disease. It is Alzheimer's disease.

Every year increasing numbers of elderly adults are diagnosed with this devastating disease. Statistics currently reveal that 10 percent of people over the age of 65 and 50 percent of people over the age of 85 have been diagnosed with the disorder. In the United States, over 4 million people suffer from Alzheimer's disease. Future projections are grim, estimating that by the middle of the twenty-first century, nearly 14 million will suffer from the disease.

However, although Alzheimer's disease is the most common dementia, it is not the only form of this memory-robbing disorder. Prehospital care providers need to be able to differentiate between dementia and delirium, as both conditions are found in the elderly. The purpose of this chapter is to familiarize the prehospital care provider with dementia and its progression. It will also provide information as to the nature of delirium, as EMS may be called upon to assist an elderly patient who is delirious.

DEMENTIA

Regardless of the cause, dementia is defined as a syndrome that involves the loss of memory and intellectual functioning in a way that interferes with the person's normal activities. As will be discussed later, dementia is different from delirium in its onset. Delirium has an acute onset, whereas dementia develops over a period of time. Aging alone does not cause dementia. There are several known and suspected causes of the disorder.

Dementia is not a single disease. It is a group of symptoms that accompany a clinical diagnosis or physical disorder. According to *Diagnostic and Statistic Manual of Mental Disorders,* Fourth edition (DSM-IV), in order to diagnose dementia, several criteria must exist, including:

- Short- and long-term memory impairment. The inability to retain new information or recall information from the past. Long-term memory is affected later in the disease process.
- Impaired abstract thinking. The inability to describe similarities or differences between objects.
- Impaired judgment. The inability to effectively deal with interpersonal relationships or on-the-job problems.
- Loss of higher-level brain functions resulting in conditions such as apraxia, aphasia, and agnosia.
  - Apraxia is the inability to carry out motor functions even though the patient understands those functions.
  - Aphasia is the inability to communicate by speech, in writing, or in signs. The patient may not be able to comprehend spoken or written communications.
  - Agnosia is the inability to recognize familiar objects or people.
- A change in the patient's personality. Often the change is from docile to violent.
- These changes in mental function and behavior interfere with work or social activities.

KEY POINT

Although prehospital care providers do not diagnose dementia in the field, it is important to be aware of the diagnostic criteria.

As mentioned earlier, Alzheimer's disease is only one cause of dementia. There are four categories of dementia that affect the elderly. These four categories are Alzheimer's disease, vascular dementia (multi-infarct dementia), reversible or partially reversible dementia, and other, generally neurological, disorders.

ALZHEIMER'S DISEASE

Alzheimer's disease is also known as primary degenerative dementia, and is the most common of all forms of the disease. Approximately 50 to 60 percent of patients with dementia are diagnosed with this form of the disease. Alzheimer's disease is progressive and degenerative, not remaining stable for any prolonged period of time. The disease affects the number, structure, and function of the neurons within the brain. Although no specific cause for Alzheimer's disease has been identified, research has centered on abnormal proteins around the neurons, changes in certain chemical activities in the affected areas, viral infections, and environmental causes.

Unfortunately, the only precise way to diagnose Alzheimer's disease is by autopsy. Thus, mental health professionals diagnose Alzheimer's dementia by ruling out other causes for the dementia. In order for the diagnosis of "probable" Alzheimer's disease, certain criteria must be met, including:

- Meeting the initial criteria for dementia (see earlier discussion of dementia).
- Age of onset between 40 and 90 years of age.
- No signs, symptoms, or evidence of systemic or brain disease.
- One or more deficits in cognition such as apraxia, aphasia, and agnosia.
- Gradual worsening of memory and cognitive functions.
- As the disease progresses, there are certain clinical features that add to the diagnosis of Alzheimer's disease. These features include:
  - A leveling off in the progress of the disease for up to 2 years.
  - Clinical findings of insomnia, bladder/bowel incontinence, delusions, hallucinations, emotional or physical outbursts, sexual disorders, and weight loss.
  - Increased muscle tone and shock-like contractions of a muscle or group of muscles (myoclonus).
  - Seizures during the advanced stage of the disease.

During the early stages of the disease, patients will complain of forgetfulness, often characterized by misplacing commonly used items and repeating words or activities. This should not be interpreted to mean that simple forgetfulness such as misplacing car keys is an indication of dementia! Most people in the early stage of Alzheimer's disease are aware that something is wrong, and refer themselves to their doctor with mild and sometimes vague complaints. Occasionally, the prehospital care provider may respond to a call that involves a patient who may be suffering from the early stage of Alzheimer's disease. Although most patients undergo a quick assessment to determine orientation to time, person, place, and date, a more detailed evaluation of the elderly patient can increase the index of suspicion for Alzheimer's disease.

KEY POINT

Patients in the early stages of Alzheimer's dementia will be forgetful, and may not remember where they live or how they got to where they were found.

If the prehospital care provider suspects dementia, a short test can be given to determine the patient's mental status. There are many standardized tests found in the literature; however, some of those tests may be too detailed for prehospital care use. One such test is the Folstein Mini Mental State Examination. It is rather thorough and time consuming, so its use in prehospital care is not recommended. The following questionnaire is a quick and relatively easy-to-use test developed by the authors of *Essentials of Clinical Geriatrics* called the Short Portable Mental Status Questionnaire. This test presents 10 questions and the patient receives a point for each wrong answer.

Short Portable Mental Status Questionnaire

Right	Wrong	
_____	_____	What is the date today (month/day/year)?
_____	_____	What day of the week is it?
_____	_____	What is the name of this place?
_____	_____	What is your telephone number? (If none, ask address.)
_____	_____	How old are you?
_____	_____	When were you born (month/day/year)?
_____	_____	Who is the current president of the United States?
_____	_____	What was your mother's maiden name?
_____	_____	Subtract 3 from 20 and continue until you get all the way down.

Scoring: 0–2 errors—Intact
3–4 errors—Mild intellectual impairment
5–7 errors—Moderate intellectual impairment
8–10 errors—Severe intellectual impairment

Another quick mental status examination used by some EMS agencies is the Folstein Mini Mental Status Examination. The questions/assessments/tasks can be placed onto a card or single sheet of paper that the prehospital care provider can use to administer the examination. Like the Short Portable Mental Status Questionnaire, points are assigned to each component and are totaled after the examination has been completed.

If dementia is suspected, alert the emergency department staff so that they may conduct a more thorough evaluation of the patient.

KEY POINT

A Mini Mental Status Examination can be administered in the field and is an extension of the brief mental state questions used to determine a patient's orientation to person, place, and time.

As Alzheimer's disease progresses, the forgetfulness worsens and it begins to interfere with work or activities of daily living. At work, the employee may forget to complete an important project or may be unable to take care of a company's financial record keeping. This could place the employee's job in jeopardy. At home, the patient may have difficulty keeping up with or managing their own financial affairs, becoming delinquent in paying bills. The patient

The Folstein Mini Mental Status Examination – Part 1

Patient Name: _____   Date _____

Patient's Age: _____   Patient's Sex: _____

___/5 What is the (year) (season) (date) (day) (month)?

___/5 Where are we? (state) (country) (town) (building) (floor)

___/3 Learn: "apple, table, penny." _____ # of trials

___/5 Subtract serial 7s: (100, 93, 86, 79, 72) or spell "WORLD" backward.

___/3 Recall: "apple, table, penny."

___/2 Name "pencil" and "watch."

___/2 Repeat: "No ifs, ands, or buts."

___/3 "Take this paper in your right hand, fold it in half, and put it on the floor."

___/1 Read and obey: "Close your eyes." (see back of card)

___/1 Write a sentence on the back of this card.

___/1 Copy the design on the back of this card.

___/30 Total (Abnormal is < 24 or if < 8th grade, then < 21 is abnormal.)

The Folstein Mini Mental Status Examination – Part 2

Close your eyes

_____

Source: Folstein Fetal & Psychiatric Res, 1975. This tool is widely available on the Internet and is also available for downloading for use on a hand-held (PDA) device.

may forget to take their medications or may wander from home, forgetting where they live or how to return there. Eventually, the patient with Alzheimer's disease will be unable to care for him or herself.

Our discussion has primarily centered on the initial stages of Alzheimer's disease. However, there are four stages of the disease, each one progressively worse than the one before. During the first stage of the disease, the patient may

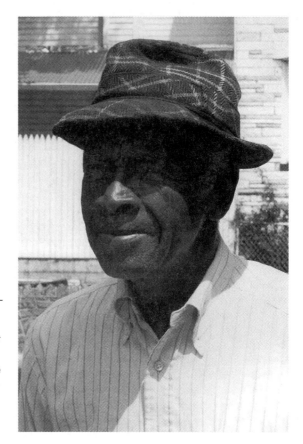

• FIGURE 5-1
In the early stages of Alzheimer's disease memory disturbances are prominent.

Source: From *Aging,* a magazine of the Administration on Aging, www.aoa.dhhs.gov/aoa/ magimage/magimage.html.

notice that something is wrong without being sure exactly what is amiss. The patient may be depressed or anxious. Memory disturbances are the most prominent complaint. As the initial stage progresses, the patient may also complain of not being able to solve problems, especially if the problem is complex. For example, the patient may not be able to balance a checkbook or prepare a complex meal. The patient's abstract thoughts and ability to make critical decisions are also impaired.

As the patient enters the second stage of the illness, their ability to manage business and personal affairs falters. Failing memory, decreased desire or initiative, and impaired ability to meet life's challenges are typical in this stage. Because the patient is still aware of their condition, depression or anxiety may increase.

After a period of time, the patient deteriorates and the third stage of Alzheimer's disease begins. Spontaneous speech decreases and verbal language often consists of echoing what was previously said. Written communications also deteriorate. The patient's ability to carry out simple motor skills fails, even though they may understand the skill or the request to perform that skill. The patient may be unable to identify familiar objects or faces. Occasionally, the patient seems to be acutely aware of their condition while at other times they are oblivious to it. Restlessness is common, especially in the evening (sundowning), and the patient can become very frightened even in familiar surroundings.

KEY POINT

Sundowning, or restlessness during the evening, is characteristic during the later stages of Alzheimer's dementia.

When the patient enters the final stage of Alzheimer's disease, they are no longer able to communicate. The patient may utter short phrases or may babble incoherently. Occasionally, they may involuntarily express an emotion such as laughing or crying. If friends, family, or caregivers "bother" the patient, the patient may become irritated and violent. The patient may also experience delusions. Toward the end of life, the patient becomes apathetic, withdrawn, and silent. A small percentage (10 percent) develops seizures during the last year of life. Death is the result of aspiration, pneumonia, or urinary tract infection and urosepsis.

PROBLEM BEHAVIORS SEEN IN PATIENTS WITH ALZHEIMER'S DISEASE

Although the patient's memory and intellectual functions are impaired, the patient's emotions and feelings are still intact. Occasionally, the prehospital care provider may be called to attend to someone who is displaying an abnormal behavior that seems inappropriate. The patient with Alzheimer's disease cannot control their emotions and, therefore may display any number of problem behaviors that attract the attention of law enforcement and emergency medical services. The following is a partial list of some of these abnormal behaviors.

- Repetitive and purposeless activity. The patient may be restless and tend to wander aimlessly.
- Asking the same question repeatedly.
- Shadowing a family member or caregiver.
- Hoarding or hiding things. An example is taking all the dishes and hiding them.
- Urinating or defecating in public.
- Undressing in public.
- Exposing genitals in public.
- Removing dentures in a restaurant.
- Paranoid behavior.
- Verbal or physical outbursts that could include yelling, screaming, swearing, spitting, and physical aggression.

KEY POINT

Abnormal or unusual behavior is common in the later stages of Alzheimer's dementia. Some behaviors could be considered assaultive or criminal.

MULTI-INFARCT (VASCULAR) DEMENTIA

Another major cause of dementia is multi-infarct, or small-infarct, dementia. This condition occurs when the patient has suffered a series of strokes that affect their cognitive functions. Although none of the strokes is large enough to cause residual impairment, the cumulative effect can be devastating. Although it may be difficult to differentiate between Alzheimer's disease and multi-infarct dementia, there are some distinctive findings for each disorder. Multi-infarct dementia:

- Typically strikes more men than women.
- Progresses sporadically, usually after a subsequent stroke.

- Is seen more frequently in patients with a history of hypertension.
- Shows evidence of prior strokes, TIAs, or focal neurological signs such as hemiparesis, hemiplegia, gait abnormalities, or the exaggeration of deep tendon reflexes.

OTHER CAUSES OF DEMENTIA

Some causes of dementia are reversible and others are partially reversible. The mnemonic DEMENTIA has been developed to help identify some of the potentially reversible causes of dementia. Please remember that the dementia may remain even after the suspected cause has been treated or removed. DEMENTIA stands for the following:

D	Drugs
E	Emotional disorders
M	Metabolic or endocrine disorders
E	Eye and ear disorders
N	Nutritional deficiencies
T	Tumors and trauma
I	Infections
A	Arteriosclerotic complications

There are several other neurological conditions that can lead to a demented state. These other irreversible causes include Parkinson's disease and Huntington's chorea.

KEY POINT

Some causes of dementia are reversible. When the cause is removed, the dementia may resolve.

DISTINGUISHING DELIRIUM FROM DEMENTIA

Delirium is often confused with dementia. Prehospital care providers should be able to differentiate between the two conditions as there are several unique differences between them.

Delirium is defined as an acute transient change in a patient's mental status. It is accompanied by a change in consciousness and cognition. According to DSM-IV, there are certain distinguishing features of delirium. These features include:

- Prompt onset of the signs and symptoms, often in a matter of hours or days.
- Decreased ability to pay attention to external stimuli. When performing patient assessment, the same questions have to be asked repeatedly.
- Disorganized thinking that may be characterized by disorganized or rambling speech.

- Reduced level of consciousness.
- Misperception of surroundings, illusions, or hallucinations.
- Difficulty in recognizing time, person, or place.
- Impaired memory.

KEY POINT

Delirium differs from dementia in several aspects, such as its quick onset and the patient's disorganized thoughts and reduced level of consciousness.

Many causes of delirium are reversible; however, resolving the cause does not guarantee the resolution of the delirium. Some causes of delirium in the elderly include:

- Malnutrition
- Hypoxia (too little oxygen in the blood)
- Hypercapnia (too much carbon dioxide in the blood)
- Blood sugar imbalances (too much or too little)
- Some medications
- Alcohol abuse
- Infections
- Depression
- Dehydration
- Stroke
- Heat or cold emergencies
- Fecal impaction
- Urinary retention

In caring for the older adult with suspected delirium, if the underlying cause is identified and treated, the delirium may abate.

To help differentiate delirium from dementia, ask the patient's family members or caregivers if the change in behavior was sudden or if the abnormal behavior developed over a prolonged period of time. Again, the onset of delirium is quick, over hours to days, as opposed to dementia, which may progress over months to years.

SOME THOUGHTS ABOUT BENIGN SENESCENT FORGETFULNESS

Another common condition that can be confused with dementia is benign senescent forgetfulness (formerly known as senility).

Although benign senescent forgetfulness involves varying degrees of memory loss, it does not progress and does not interfere with daily living. Typically, the patient's repetition of questions or memories of events characterizes the condition. At first glance, it appears the patient may have dementia. The only way to make a differential diagnosis is to observe the patient for several months, watching for any deterioration in condition.

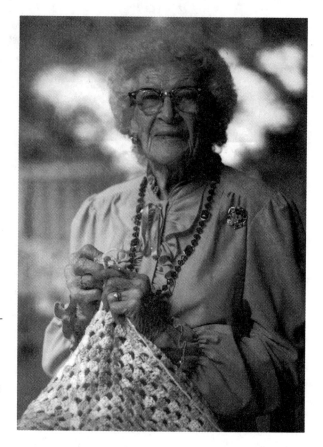

• FIGURE 5-2
Benign forgetfulness can be
disconcerting to the older
adult.

Source: From *Aging,* a magazine
of the Administration on Aging,
www.aoa.dhhs.gov/aoa/
magimage/magimage.html.

KEY POINT

Most people occasionally forget things. This does not indicate dementia.

THE EMS ROLE IN ALZHEIMER'S DISEASE

Although prehospital care providers will generally not be involved in the daily care of the patient with Alzheimer's disease, prehospital care providers may be called to assist in the search for a patient who has wandered and become lost or if the patient is injured. An EMS response may also be necessary if the Alzheimer's patient becomes verbally or physically abusive.

At times, EMS may be summoned to attend to a person who seems to be lost and disoriented. When on such calls, the prehospital care provider must be alert to the possibility of Alzheimer's disease and look for any of the following signs or symptoms.

- Over- or underdressed.
- Seems to be absentminded.
- Has difficulty responding to simple questions.
- Asks for the same information repeatedly.
- Seems to have impaired judgment.
- Is disoriented.
- Is unable to talk.
- Is unable to follow directions.

There will be times when EMS responds to a patient with known Alzheimer's disease. To help assess the patient and expedite patient care, the prehospital care provider should keep these key concepts in mind.

- Talk slowly. Aging slows the patient's ability to process information. In patients with Alzheimer's disease, this process can be even slower. Some patients may not be able to process the information at all. Ask questions slowly and wait for responses. If necessary, repeat the question.
- Establish and maintain eye contact. This helps to reassure a frightened patient.
- Ask caregivers, family members, and friends for important information.
- Watch for and be prepared to handle aggressive or assaultive behavior. Patients with Alzheimer's disease may have difficulty with simple tasks such as dressing or feeding themselves. This can be frustrating, and patients may strike out verbally or physically. Some patients become intimidated by strange or new sounds. Silence loud noises, reduce extraneous sounds such as the dispatch radio, and have one person communicate with the patient.

If the patient becomes physically assaultive, there are several steps the prehospital care provider can take prior to placing the patient into restraints. These steps include:

- Ask the patient to stop the behavior. Be specific in identifying the behavior. Merely stating "Stop that" will probably have no effect.
- Redirect the patient. Try to redirect the patient's attention to another matter. Instructing the patient to "Get your glasses" or "Get your hearing aid" can put the agitated patient onto a different path—one of cooperation. As the patient calms, enter into a verbal agreement with the patient to discontinue the unwanted behavior.
- Use the "Rule of 5s." The Rule of 5s means using no more than five words per sentence with no more than five letters per word. Long, complex sentences that consist of long words with multiple syllables are confusing to the Alzheimer's patient. For example, say, "Don't throw your food," as opposed to, "If you don't stop throwing your food, we'll have to restrain you."
- Reassure the patient. Let the patient know that he or she is safe and secure.

If these techniques fail, it may become necessary to physically restrain the combative patient.

DOWN THE ROAD—THE FUTURE

There is no known cure for Alzheimer's disease. Researchers have tried to isolate a specific cause for the disorder and have identified some treatments that alleviate or stabilize the condition. In the 1970s, some researchers discovered that Alzheimer's patients had a reduced amount of acetylcholine, a neurotransmitter, in the nerve synapses. Additional research focused on the idea that the disease interferes with the production of this chemical or the chemical that destroys it (cholinesterase).

Two drugs were developed that block cholinesterase production, thus increasing the amount of acetylcholine in the brain. These two drugs, Cognex (tacrine) and Aricept (donepezil), have been shown to slow the progress of the disease, but not cure it. Recent studies have shown that tacrine only benefits 20 to 40 percent of the patients who take the medication. Tacrine is costly and has severe side effects, including nausea and vomiting, along with an increased chance of liver disease. Liver enzymes increase significantly in patients taking tacrine.

Donepezil is better tolerated by Alzheimer's patients. Patients taking this medication have shown improvement in cognitive and motor skills. Although donepezil can also cause nausea and vomiting, its effects on liver enzymes are less than those of tacrine. Like the other medications used to treat Alzheimer's disease, donepezil is expensive.

There are other cholinesterase inhibitors under review, including Promem (metrifonate), rivastigmin, and galantamine, that have shown great promise in clinical trials.

Other forms of therapy for Alzheimer's disease include estrogen therapy, calcium channel blockers, and antioxidant vitamins such as vitamins A, C, and E. Some alternative forms of therapy have also been reviewed. Ginkgo biloba, an over-the-counter herbal remedy has been shown to enhance memory and cognitive function. In Europe, particularly in Germany, ginkgo biloba has been endorsed as therapy for Alzheimer's disease.

SUMMARY

Dementia is a devastating disease that commonly affects the elderly. Prehospital care providers will be called upon to care for patients with this debilitating condition and need to be aware of the progression of the illness and its ultimate effects.

The patient with Alzheimer's will not recover. The patient will continue to deteriorate and lose their memory and intellectual functioning. The patient may wander away from home, become lost, sustain injuries, and require prehospital intervention.

Prehospital care providers may also encounter patients who are delirious. By recognizing delirium and looking for its underlying causes, the prehospital care provider can begin care that could reverse or resolve the condition.

Regardless of the nature or cause of memory loss, prehospital care providers must display a high level of compassion for these older adults.

ON THE JOB

You are called to a city park where you are greeted by a police officer who tells you that a 78-year-old woman is "acting funny and I think we should restrain her." She is standing next to the park's restroom building, clutching her purse, and saying that she is looking for Ed's Market. The officer tells you that Ed's Market closed 20 years ago. Describe your initial approach to the patient. If, after talking to the woman, she becomes combative, describe how you would calm the patient in order to keep her safe and provide care.

Elder Abuse—The Silent Cry

OBJECTIVES

At the end of the chapter, the reader will be able to:

1 Define elder abuse as physical abuse, neglect, intimidation, cruel punishment, fiduciary abuse, abandonment, or other treatment resulting in pain or physical or mental suffering.

2 List the five types of abuse seen in elder abuse cases.

3 Describe physical abuse.

4 Discuss how failure to obtain medical care is an indication of physical abuse.

5 Discuss how overmedication is an indication of physical abuse, especially when the medication is used as a chemical restraint.

6 Define fiduciary abuse as a form of elder abuse.

7 Define psychological abuse as a form of elder abuse.

8 Define violation of rights as a form of elder abuse.

9 Define neglect as a form of elder abuse.

10 List the two general causes of elder abuse as internal stress and external stress.

11 List 10 characteristics of the abuse victim.

12 List nine characteristics of the abuser.

13 Discuss what information should be documented pertaining to the suspicion of elder abuse.

14 Describe what the right of self-determination means.

WORDS TO KNOW

Abuse   Physical abuse, neglect, intimidation, cruel punishment, fiduciary abuse, abandonment, or other treatment resulting in pain or physical or mental suffering.

Chemical restraint   The use of medications to sedate and control a person.

Coercion   To dominate or bring about by threat or force.

Conservatorship   To place a person under guardianship.

Decubitus ulcer   Damage to the skin and underlying structures by pressure. A bedsore.

Durable power of attorney   A legal document conferring authority to act as attorney or agent for someone.

Ecchymosis   Black and blue discoloration as seen in bruising.

Fiduciary abuse   Misuse of funds or property that belong to another person. Theft.

Neglect   Failure to provide food, clothing, or shelter.

Psychological abuse   Verbal assaults or threats that create fear.

In Chapter 1 of this book, we looked at the increasing number of elderly in the United States. With a blossoming older adult population, there are increasing demands to provide health care and living arrangements. Often, caring for the elderly falls upon the family, and family members may be unprepared for the added responsibilities of caring for an aging and often infirm parent. The end result is elder abuse—a new and increasing form of societal violence.

Prehospital care providers are increasingly called upon to assist the elderly. Often the initial contact with the healthcare profession begins with the call to 9-1-1. Prehospital care providers can be vital in identifying elder abuse that could otherwise go unnoticed.

Some states require prehospital care providers to report elder abuse when they observe an actual incident, discover physical injury caused by abuse, or are told of abuse by the victim. The abuse does not have to be actual physical violence. There are a number of forms of abuse the prehospital care provider may see.

Along with the requirement to report elder abuse, some states impose criminal penalties such as fines and/or imprisonment for failure to report abuse. For example, in California, failure to report elder abuse is a misdemeanor punishable by up to 6 months in jail and/or a $1,000 fine. Additionally, prehospital care providers may also lose their certification.

KEY POINT

Elder abuse is becoming increasingly common and many states require prehospital care providers to report suspected abuse or face fines or imprisonment or both.

The purpose of this chapter is to familiarize the prehospital care provider with the various forms of elder abuse, including physical abuse, fiduciary abuse, psychological abuse, violation of rights, and neglect. Although the pre-hospital care provider may not see all forms of abuse, the provider should be aware of all the different types of abuse.

This chapter will also address the common causes of abuse, such as internal and external stresses, and describe the type of person who would abuse the elderly. A profile of the abused victim will also be presented.

Additionally, the chapter will present information on the procedures to follow when elder abuse is suspected, as well as the information that needs to be documented and reported. Finally, guidelines for intervention with the abuse victim will be discussed. Being prepared to assess and intervene in elder abuse situations may prevent the untimely death of a senior and help the victim return to a productive or reasonable quality of life.

TYPES OF ELDER ABUSE

Abuse is defined as physical abuse, neglect, intimidation, cruel punishment, fiduciary abuse, abandonment, or other treatment resulting in pain or physical or mental suffering. Depriving the person of goods or services that are necessary to avoid physical harm or mental suffering is also abuse. Elder abuse is, for all purposes, similar to child abuse; however, with elder abuse there is the addition of financial or fiduciary abuse not typically seen in child abuse.

There are five types of abuse: physical, fiduciary, psychological, rights violations, and neglect. Each type of abuse has specific signs associated with the abuse.

PHYSICAL ABUSE

Physical abuse consists of direct physical harm such as injuries from domestic violence. Key indicators of physical abuse include:

- Signs of physical injury such as scratches, bruises, cuts, burns, or traumatic alopecia
- Restraint injuries
- Use of chemical restraint
- Repeated, unexplained, or hidden injuries
- Doctor/emergency department shopping (i.e., finding a doctor who will give the desired drugs or not notice unusual complaints or physical findings)
- Time lags between injury and treatment

Unusual bruises or injuries that do not match the description of how the injury occurred should be viewed with suspicion. Ecchymosis around the eye or a black eye could be caused by accidental blunt trauma or an intentionally inflicted blow to the face. Ask how the bruise appeared and what was done to treat it. Cigarette burns or circumferential abrasions around the wrists or ankles caused by restraints should also arouse suspicion. Be suspicious if the patient is missing large chunks of hair from the hair being forcibly pulled.

KEY POINT

Be suspicious of injuries that do not match the description of the cause. Intentionally inflicted injuries are often glossed over by the victim or the abuser.

Because of the aging process and changes in the skin, the older adult is more likely to develop pressure sores (decubitus ulcers) on certain areas of the body. The usual sites for decubitus ulcers include the coccyx (tailbone), buttocks, heels, and elbows, or any location that is in constant contact with a firm surface. The initial appearance of the injury is reddening of the skin. With continued pressure, it can rapidly worsen, forming an ulcer. The worst stage of decubitus ulcer (Stage IV) includes ulceration and damage to muscle and, perhaps, the exposure of bone. (See Chapter 8, Medical Emergencies, for more specific information on decubitus ulcers.)

Decubitus ulcers can develop from lying in one position for extended periods of time. If the prehospital care provider encounters a decubitus ulcer, it should be cared for in a manner similar to any other injury. However, note the location and appearance of the ulceration. Also note the bedding and the patient's surroundings. The mere presence of a decubitus ulcer does not indicate elder abuse. However, the presence of a decubitus ulcer accompanied by unsanitary conditions and, perhaps, an uncooperative family might indicate abuse.

KEY POINT

Assessing a bed-ridden older patient for decubitus ulcers is essential. Look for decubitus ulcers on the feet, heels, ankles, buttocks, hips, and back.

Failure to obtain or delays in obtaining medical care is an indication of physical abuse. For example, the prehospital care providers may strongly urge that the patient be taken to the emergency department. Yet, the family or caregivers insist on transporting the patient to the hospital or doctor's office "in a

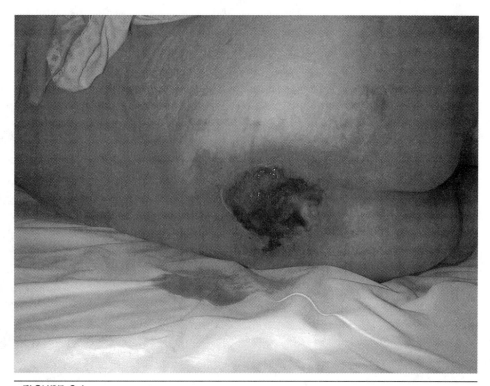

• FIGURE 6-1
Stage IV decubitus ulcer on the sacrum.
Courtesy of Charles Stewart, MD FACEP; www.storysmith.net

while." Hours or days pass and EMS is again summoned to the scene to find the patient in the same or worse condition because the family or caregivers failed to obtain medical care for the patient.

Overmedication or failure to follow the medication regimen can also be viewed as physical abuse. Giving the patient too much of a necessary medication increases the risk of an overdose. If the patient is known to be depressed, a caregiver may give the patient an additional dose of antidepressants to elevate the patient's mood for some self-serving interest. More common, though, is the excessive use of medications as a chemical restraint. Giving the elderly patient an extra dose of sleeping pills or a mild tranquilizer to keep the patient under control is considered physical abuse.

KEY POINT

Physical and chemical restraint are often used by abusive caregivers to keep the victim "under control."

Not only are chemical restraints used to control the elderly, physical restraints are also used to keep the patient in bed or in a wheelchair. Although some patients need physical restraints to keep from injuring themselves, these restraints are to be used only on the advice of a physician—in other words, restraints require a prescription. The typical restraints seen in the hospital setting are not available to the average citizen. Therefore, a caregiver may improvise, using sheets, towels, ropes, or chains to restrain the older person. For example, one elderly woman was found in an aluminum shed restrained to her bed with chains.

At times the abuser will use physical restraint to punish the older adult. Out of frustration, the abusive family member or caregiver ties the patient to their bed, admonishing the patient for some usually trivial wrongdoing. Addi-

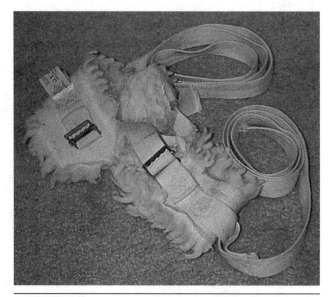

• FIGURE 6-2
Fabric restraints are used to restrict arm and leg movement, as well as help confine a patient to bed.

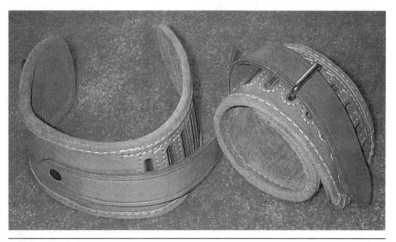

• FIGURE 6-3
Look for fabric or leather restraints that may be attached to a bed or wheelchair.

tionally, the caregiver may punish the patient by refusing to give the person food or water. Failure to provide adequate hydration or nutrition to a person can lead to dehydration and malnutrition or worsen an existing condition.

Finally, physical abuse can also consist of sexual exploitation. Prehospital care providers will rarely encounter this form of abuse; however, some elderly are raped or sodomized by the caregiver.

FIDUCIARY ABUSE

Prehospital care providers rarely see fiduciary abuse. However, an elderly patient might describe fiduciary abuse to the prehospital care provider while they are being transported to the emergency department. Types of fiduciary abuse include:

- Theft
- Misuse of funds
- Extortion
- Fraud
- Phone scams
- Phony sweepstakes

Fiduciary or financial abuse typically consists of theft from the older adult. The elder adult could be the victim of a financial scam by an unknown person. For example, a person may approach the older adult and tell them about sharing in some recently found money, but the older adult first needs to contribute to the funds. The unsuspecting elderly withdraws a significant sum of money from the bank and entrusts it to the other person. After waiting for the "payoff," the senior realizes that the money and the hopes for riches have vanished.

Misuse of funds or property is another type of fiduciary abuse. For example, an elderly woman entrusts her family with her money, hoping to be cared for during her old age. Unfortunately, the family spends the money for personal gain, and, after a short time, the bank accounts are depleted.

Some elderly are asked to assign property rights to a family member so that the property can be maintained. Sadly, in some cases the family member or caregiver sells the property and takes the money.

If the prehospital care provider hears the elderly patient complain that their family has taken all of their money, the prehospital care provider should consider reporting it to the appropriate authorities for investigation. Granted, the patient may have dementia; however, it is best to inform the emergency department or state agency of potential fiduciary abuse.

PSYCHOLOGICAL ABUSE

Psychological abuse consists of a living environment that creates fear. Psychological abuse often includes:

- Verbal assaults
- Threats
- Creation of fear
- Isolation
- Withholding of support

Intimidation through threats to cause harm prevents the abuse victim from reporting any physical abuse. This is also found in child abuse where the abuser tells the victim not to say anything to anyone or there will be more physical punishment.

Psychological abuse may include the isolation of the victim from anyone who may be able to report the abuse. Isolation should not be confused with being alone or lonely. Isolation is deliberately preventing the older adult from seeing friends or other family members in an attempt to control the person and to protect the caregiver.

KEY POINT

Watch for intimidation by the caregiver. It can be subtle.

The withholding of emotional support is also considered psychological abuse. When the victim needs to be consoled due to a loss or other stressful event, the abusive caregiver refuses to give emotional support. Emotional support could be as simple as a smile or a hug or as much as empathic listening. The caregiver punishes the patient by withholding any support.

When assessing an older patient who may be the victim of psychological abuse, be alert for:

- Ambivalence
- Anxiety
- Depression or hopelessness
- Trembling
- Clinging
- Cowering
- Lack of eye contact
- Agitation or hypervigilance

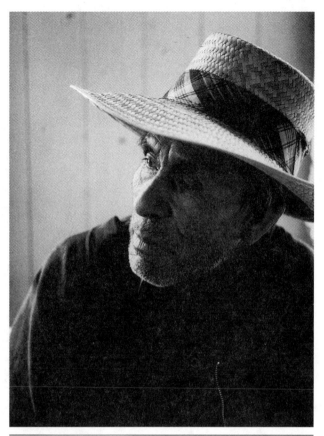

• FIGURE 6-4

Look for subtle signs of elder abuse.

Source: From *Aging,* a magazine from the Administration on Aging, www.aoa.dhhs.gov/aoa/magimage/magimage.html.

VIOLATION OF RIGHTS

Violation of rights is another form of elder abuse. Violation of rights involves:

- Coercion
- Locking up the victim in a room
- Abandonment
- Forced removal from home

Coercion is defined as control through suggestion or domination. In other words, to bully the elderly person into doing something that they would not normally do. Coercion may not be overt at the scene of an emergency call. Watch for facial or body expressions that indicate intimidation or coercion. If the patient attempts to say something and suddenly stops, consider that there may be a reason, such as coercion, for the silence.

Look for locks on the outside of the victim's bedroom. Locking the patient into their room is a violation of the person's rights, especially if it interferes with the activities of daily living and could result in harm.

If the victim is left alone at home for prolonged periods without food or water, the victim may have been abandoned. This could occur if the caregiver is required to work in order to care for the older adult. When the caregiver is working, the elderly person may be locked into a room without food or water for several hours.

Forceful ejection of an elderly person from their home or place of residence may be the result of fiduciary abuse where the family or caregiver has sold or lost the victim's property. Occasionally, the courts can intervene and delay a forced eviction.

In some cities where rent control is in effect, landlords are prevented from significantly raising the rent unless the tenant leaves the residence. Some landlords have opted to eject a tenant, usually for fabricated or flimsy reasons, in order to raise the rent and increase profits.

NEGLECT

Neglect is the failure to provide food, clothing, or shelter for the elderly. It can also be the failure to provide for their health and safety, as well as not providing for their medical care. The prehospital care provider witnesses neglect if the patient is found in unsafe or unsanitary conditions and has been deprived of food and water. Report any suspicions of neglect to the appropriate authorities as soon as possible.

COMMON CAUSES OF ELDER ABUSE

There are two general causes of elder abuse—internal stress and external stress. The abuser reacts differently to each stressor, internal and external, sometimes lashing out against the victim in anger. At other times, the abuser reacts to the stress in a quiet and subdued way, taking steps to avoid the stress, usually by physically abusing, verbally controlling, or coercing the victim.

Everyone faces stress. It is how a person copes with that stress that can pave the way for abuse. Internal stress is primarily seen as anxiety caused by relationship problems with the older adult. As a person gets older, the person may have increasing demands for care from the family member or caregiver. Greater demands for time and care can create resentment in the caregiver, who may then abuse the victim physically or psychologically.

What could increase the risk of elder abuse is a pattern of childhood abuse suffered by the caregiver. A caregiver who was abused as a child may be more likely to abuse the abusive parent when that parent becomes frail. The elder may have been a victim of abuse by a spouse.

Domestic violence by spouses can lead to continued violence and abuse later in life. A woman who was a victim of domestic violence early in her marriage is likely to be a victim later in life.

As children, we depend upon our parents for support, relying upon them for food, clothing, shelter, and the essentials of daily living. As an adult, we may still look to parents as providers. Thus, when it becomes necessary to take care of aged and ailing parents, the role reversal can be stressful. The adult child cannot handle the role reversal and becomes frustrated and abusive.

External stresses can also affect the caregiver. The abuser might be overwhelmed by their own physical or emotional problems. If the caregiver is unemployed or not financially sound, the stresses and frustrations caused by these problems can invite physical, psychological, and fiduciary abuse. If the caregiver is not healthy or has serious or debilitating medical conditions, the caregiver may not be able to meet the physical challenges of caring for the older adult.

External stresses of all sorts can constantly impact the caregiver. If the caregiver cannot effectively handle the stress or get some relief from it, a reaction to additional demands by a frail or sickly adult could be violent. Whenever a family member opts to care for an older adult, the older adult will eventually need continual care. Consider the aged parent with Alzheimer's disease. As the disease progresses, the demands for care, as well as the psychological upheaval within the family, can be profound. The caregiver may perceive their role as more obligatory than voluntary, eventually resenting the demands on their personal time.

PROFILES OF THE ABUSED AND THE ABUSER

The victim of abuse has characteristics that can be used as a profile, as does the abuser. Although not every abuse victim or abuser meets the criteria, the index of suspicion should increase when these characteristics are observed, especially when abuse is suspected.

The characteristics of the abuse victim include:

- Female
- Lives with the abuser
- Rarely takes action
- Compliant with the abuser
- Over 75 years of age
- Blames him or herself for the abuse
- Socially isolated from others
- Loyal to the abuser
- Frail
- Difficult behavior by the elder

In looking at the characteristics of the abuse victim, it is easy to imagine the responses the victim might give when questioned about the abuse: "It's my fault that she hit me." "I can be such a pest at times." "He is so busy at work and has little time for his mother." "I am too weak to care for myself and have no one else to care for me." "No, I don't want to press charges against him. He really is a good boy."

Similarly, the abuser has a profile—characteristics that could raise the index of suspicion if evidence of abuse is found.

The characteristics of the abuser include:

- Relative of the victim
- Drug or alcohol abuse
- Confused role
- Poor impulse control
- Involuntary caregiver
- Lives with the victim
- Externalized blame
- Displaces anger
- Lacks empathy

Keep in mind that the caregiver could be the victim's spouse, child, sibling, or hired caregiver. The caregiver often resents the victim's intrusion into their life, and blames the victim for any misfortune. If the abuser has a bad day at work, it is the victim's fault: "I was so upset worrying about you, that I couldn't get my work done." The abuser displaces anger onto the victim and strikes out inappropriately. Because the abuser cannot control their impulses, the abuser will use physical violence as an answer to their external and internal stresses. The abuser has no knowledge about, and does not care, to empathize with the health decline or concerns of the older adult.

GUIDELINES FOR ASSESSMENT AND DOCUMENTATION

When the prehospital care provider suspects elder abuse, the provider needs to fully assess the situation and carefully document any findings. The patient care report can be used in court if elder abuse is confirmed.

In an emergency, it will not be possible to adhere to all of the following guidelines. Each situation will vary depending upon the patient's condition and the environment surrounding the incident. The prehospital care provider should use proper judgment in determining which guidelines can be implemented at the time of the call.

Whenever possible, interview the victim alone. This may not be possible while on the scene and preparing to transport the patient. However, while transporting the patient to the emergency department, it may be possible to interview the victim without the interference of the abuser.

Document all information, including the patient's statements, using direct quotes when possible. Do not accuse the abuser or make suggestions to the victim that they were abused. Do not make such statements in your report. Allow the patient to tell their story. Report any other relevant information, such as the physical surroundings at the scene. Once the patient is turned over to the staff at the emergency department, speak to the physician or other appropriate staff about your suspicions. Some states require a written report within 2 days of the incident. Be sure to follow state or local laws when reporting suspected elder abuse.

If time permits, submit a comprehensive report. The following guidelines are only suggestions. Do not delay patient care or transportation to the hospital to obtain this information.

A comprehensive report should document the patient's functional level, including their ability to perform activities of daily living such as dressing, feeding, and bathing. If it can be determined, state how dependent the elderly person is on the caregiver. Also include such information as the names of the caregivers, where they live in relation to the victim, and how often the victim sees the caregivers.

Document the urgency of the situation. Is the situation one that requires an immediate response from a state or local agency? Is there a high level of risk to the victim's personal health and safety? If a medical emergency exists, provide immediate care and transportation to the emergency department. If a physical assault is occurring at the time of arrival, be sure to request a police response if they are not already en route. If the situation is nonemergent, document the situation and make sure that follow-up is suggested.

> ### KEY POINT
>
> Thoroughly document all findings, including the patient's statements and objective findings such as the patient's functional level and the urgency of the situation.

INTERVENTION ISSUES

If the prehospital care provider has to intervene in an abusive situation, it is usually to stop the abuse from continuing and to provide medical care to the victim at the scene and while en route to the emergency department. There are some basics to keep in mind when assisting the older adult in an abusive situation.

First, there is the issue of confidentiality. The victim has the right to privacy. Whenever possible and appropriate, obtain consent from the patient to report the incident to the authorities. If the patient is mentally competent, they have the right to refuse any unwanted intrusion. There are four levels of mental status to be considered.

> ### KEY POINT
>
> The patient has the right to privacy. Maintain confidentiality.

The first level of mental status is when the patient is mentally clear, understands what has happened, and is willing to accept the care and intervention that has been offered.

The second level of mental status is when the patient is mentally clear, understands what has happened, but does not accept the offer of care and intervention. The patient will not cooperate with anyone regarding the abuse.

A third level of mental status is when the patient has been determined to be incapable of making their own decisions by court action. In these cases, the patient may have been placed into a conservatorship by the court. The conservator must be contacted regarding the abuse. The patient's mental status is not an issue during a life-threatening medical emergency. Most states use the concept of implied consent to provide for the medical treatment of disease or injury at the scene of an emergency.

Finally, a fourth level exists when the patient lacks the ability to make a clinical decision, but has not been determined incompetent by court action. In some cases, the patient's caregivers may have a signed durable power of attorney giving them the right to determine the nature and level of care to be given to the patient.

It is important to remember that the patient has the right to self-determination. The patient has the right to make all decisions regarding their care unless they have given that authority to someone else or the courts have appointed someone to make those decisions. Freedom is, at times, more important than safety. A person can choose to live in harm or self-destruction if they are competent to make that choice, and their choice does not harm others or break the law.

KEY POINT

The patient has the right of self-determination and can accept or reject any offer of help.

SUMMARY

Elder abuse is increasingly becoming a problem. With a growing number of older adults and diminishing resources to provide care, many elderly are turning to their family for assistance. With increasing care demands on the family and stresses on family relationships, the possibility of elder abuse is great.

The prehospital care provider will encounter evidence of elder abuse. Abuse such as physical injury, psychological abuse, rights violations, and neglect may be evident at the scene of the emergency. Many states have implemented laws that require prehospital care providers to report suspicions of elder abuse or face the loss of certification, a fine, and/or imprisonment.

This chapter has broached the subject of elder abuse and identified the five types of abuse. It has listed characteristics or profiles of the victim and abuser to help the prehospital care provider increase their awareness of abuse at the scene. Guidelines for documentation as well as intervention have been highlighted. Finally, the patient's right to self-determination was discussed. No matter what care or assistance is offered, it is up to the mentally competent patient to accept or reject the offer for help.

7

Pharmacology in the Older Population

OBJECTIVES

At the end of the chapter, the reader will be able to:

1 List two general forms of medications.
2 Define the following liquid forms of medications: solutions, tinctures, syrups, suspensions, spirits, emulsions, elixirs.
3 Define the following solid forms of medications: pills, powders, capsules, tablets, suppositories, ointments.
4 List nine different routes of drug administration.
5 Define the terms venous access port and venous access device.
6 Discuss why protein-bound medications may last longer in the body than medications that are not protein-bound.
7 Discuss how aging delays metabolism and excretion of a medication by the liver and kidneys.
8 State four ways that drugs can be excreted from the body.
9 Define the term compliance as it pertains to prescribed medications.
10 List six factors affecting compliance in taking prescription medications.
11 List eight factors that increase the risk for medication errors in the older adult.
12 List four types of over-the-counter medications than can adversely affect the elderly.
13 State two adverse effects of nonsteroidal anti-inflammatory drugs (NSAIDs) in the adult.
14 State six adverse effects of over-the-counter antihistamines.
15 List eight classes of medications that could cause problems in the geriatric patient.
16 Given a list of medications, match general adverse effects with the given medication.
17 Define the term tinnitus.
18 Discuss how tinnitus can interfere with the activities of daily living.
19 Understand that a number of medications can cause tinnitus in the elderly patient.
20 List seven over-the-counter herbal supplements that may be used by the older adult.
21 Understand that herbal supplements can interact with prescription medications.
22 Understand that herbal supplements can have adverse effects.

Adverse effect   Symptom or reaction caused by a medication that is harmful to a patient.

Albumin   A protein in the blood that is soluble in water. Serum albumin is an abundant protein in blood.

Anticoagulant   Drug that prevents coagulation/clotting of blood.

Antidepressant   Drug used to reverse the symptoms of depression.

Antihistamine   Drug that acts to block the effects of histamines.

Antihypertensive   Drug used to treat high blood pressure.

Brand name   Name given to a medication by its manufacturer.

Catecholamine   Group of chemicals used by the nervous system that affect heart rate, blood pressure, and other autonomic functions.

Chemical name   Name of a medication based on its chemical makeup.

Chemotherapy   Drug therapy given to cancer patients to destroy the tumors.

Compliance   Patient's adherence to the plan of therapy suggested by their physician.

Contraindications   Condition that makes the use of a particular medication undesirable or improper.

Corticosteroid   Type of hormone produced by the adrenal gland.

Dysrhythmia   Abnormal heart rhythm that may be fatal.

Gastric   Pertaining to the stomach.

Generic name   Drug name that is not protected by trademark or patent. It is based on the drug's chemical name.

Half-life   The time required for half of a medication to be metabolized and rendered ineffective in the body.

Heparin lock   Device consisting of an intravenous catheter inserted into a vein through which medications are administered intermittently.

Hyperglycemia   Excessive sugar (glucose) in the blood.

Hypoglycemia   Insufficient sugar (glucose) in the blood.

Indications   Conditions for which a drug is used.

Intramuscular injection (IM)   Giving a medication into a muscle.

Intravenous injection (IV)   Giving a medication into a vein.

Metabolite   A substance produced by metabolism; for example, when a drug is transformed from its original state by metabolism.

Monoamine oxidase   Enzyme that affects the metabolism of epinephrine and similar catecholamines.

Nebulizer   Machine that uses air or oxygen to dispense a medication in a fine mist so the patient can inhale the drug for absorption in the lungs.

Neurotransmitter   Chemical released by a nerve ending that stimulates another nerve or organ.

Nonsteroidal anti-inflammatory drugs NSAID   Drugs such as aspirin and ibuprofen that reduce inflammation.

Official name   Name given to a drug that is listed in an official registry of medications such as the United States Pharmacopoeia.

Ototoxic   Harmful or potentially damaging to the sense of hearing.

Per os (PO)   Abbreviation for the administration of a drug by mouth.

Potentiate   Enhancement of the effects of medications so that the total effect of two or more medications is more than the sum or additive effects of each drug.

Per rectum (PR)   Abbreviation for the rectal administration of a drug.

Serotonin   Neurotransmitter that stimulates smooth muscles, reduces gastric acid secretion, and produces vasoconstriction. Also plays a role in mood.

Selective serotonin reuptake inhibitor (SSRI)   Medication typically used as an antidepressant.

Side effects   Adverse effects of a medication.

Sterile abscess   A collection of fluid (usually medication) that is walled off from the tissues and cannot be absorbed by the body.

Subcutaneous (SQ and SC)   Administration of a medication under the skin.

Sublingual (SL)   Administration of a medication under the tongue.

Tinnitus   Ringing, buzzing, or roaring sound in the ears.

Topical   Administration of a medication by applying it to the skin.

Vascular access device (VAD)   A device placed in a peripheral or central vein to administer antibiotics, chemotherapy, hydration, total parenteral nutrition, or for long-term blood sampling. May be in place from 30 days to indefinitely.

Venous access port (VAP)   Plastic tube or catheter connected to a metal disc called a port. The port is implanted under the skin.

In the 1960s, the expression, "Better Living Through Chemistry" was popular. But, it merely reflected recreational drug use and did not consider prescription medications. Sadly, as we age, the body occasionally needs help regulating its functions, and it becomes necessary to take medications to prevent or treat disease.

The senior population often takes a multitude of medications—from antihypertensive medications to drugs that control the blood sugar. Most often, these medications can work together to give the patient a good quality of life. At times, however, there are adverse effects that can severely impair a person's functioning and, at times, their life.

This chapter has several purposes. This chapter will be a review of information on pharmacologic therapy. It will also provide information on medications that may pose a problem for the older adult, such as those with severe adverse effects and those that might interfere with the quality of life of the senior citizen. Information will also be presented on medications that affect hearing, especially those that can cause tinnitus. Finally, the chapter will discuss a few of the herbal remedies that some older adults are using to enhance their lives.

BACK TO BASICS

Drug Forms

This section reviews the available forms of medications. The older adult, depending on their physical status and drug needs, may take any one of several drug forms—from pill to ointment to inhaler. Medications are derived from a variety of sources and are available in a number of different forms. In prehospital care, EMS will often give the liquid form of a drug during an emergency. Yet, most people self-administer medications in some sort of solid form; for example, taking a pill.

Medications come in two general forms: liquids and solids. There are a variety of forms within each category. Prehospital care providers will encounter a variety of drug forms and they should be familiar with the nature of these forms of medication.

Liquid drugs primarily consist of a powered medication that is dissolved or mixed in a solution of water or other liquid. The powder or solid form of the medication is called the solute and the liquid portion of the drug is called the solvent. Various liquid forms of medication include:

- **Solutions.** Form of medication where powdered drugs are dissolved in water or other solvent. Solutions are generally clear. Some solutions are administered by injection whereas others are given by aerosol sprays. Aerosols can consist of a dissolved powder or a spirit that is combined with a propellant and inhaled. People with insulin-dependent diabetes use a solution containing insulin that is kept refrigerated.
- **Tinctures.** Form of medication where drugs are extracted or removed from their sources by alcohol. Some residual alcohol remains with the tincture.
- **Suspensions.** These are drugs that do not dissolve in liquid. A powdered form of a drug is mixed with a liquid, but, if left standing, the drug will separate and sink to the bottom of the liquid. Suspensions include liniments and lotions that are applied topically.
- **Spirits.** These are drugs that are mixed with a liquid that quickly evaporates (spirit). Drugs that are dissolved in or mixed in alcohol are known as spirits. The alcohol base may have an adverse effect on the patient's mental status.
- **Emulsions.** Form of medication where drugs are mixed with a liquid that cannot dissolve it, usually an oily substance. When the emulsion is shaken, globules of "fat" float on the surface. Creams are emulsions that are applied topically. Some emulsions must be refrigerated. Therefore, EMS crews should ask about medications kept in the refrigerator.
- **Elixirs.** These are alcohol-based drugs to which flavorings or sweeteners have been added to enhance palatability. Like spirits, the alcohol may have an adverse effect on the patient's level of consciousness.
- **Syrups.** Form of medication where drugs are dissolved in a sugar-water base to make them taste better.

Solid drugs are found in several forms that include:

- **Pills.** Form of solid drug where powdered drugs are compressed and shaped into a form that is easy to swallow. Often, pills are coated to prevent them from dissolving in the mouth or to make swallowing easier.
- **Powders.** These are drugs that remain in powdered form. Powders can be mixed with foods such as applesauce, enabling the older adult to swallow the medication.
- **Capsules.** Form of solid medication where powdered drugs are packaged in a container that dissolves in the body. The container, usually gelatin, is easily swallowed and dissolves in the gastrointestinal tract.
- **Tablets.** These are powdered drugs compressed into a round disk or other flattened shape.
- **Suppositories.** A form of solid drug where drugs are mixed into a compound that is solid at room temperature, but that dissolves when

exposed to the higher temperature inside the body. Once inserted rectally or vaginally, the suppository dissolves and the body absorbs the drug. Some people, young and old, are unfamiliar with suppositories and have mistakenly ingested them.

- **Ointments.** These are medications in a semisolid base that are applied to the skin for protection, as an astringent, or as a medication to be gradually absorbed through the skin. For example, nitroglycerin may be applied to the skin in an ointment form.

KEY POINT

Look around the patient's residence for various forms of medication. Make sure to look in a variety of locations, including the medicine cabinet and the refrigerator.

Getting There

In order to be therapeutic, a drug has to enter the body and it has to be transported to the site(s) of action. Thus, the speed at which a drug begins its activity initially depends on its rate of absorption into the bloodstream. Once a drug is absorbed, its effectiveness depends on its distribution through the body. Finally, a medication's efficacy is affected by metabolism and excretion.

In this section we will examine several factors that affect the absorption rate of a drug into the bloodstream. These factors include the route of administration, dosage, and form of the medication.

Depending on the type of medication and the desired speed of effect, there are several routes of administration by which drugs can be self-administered. These routes of administration include the following: intravenous (IV), intramuscular (IM), subcutaneous (SC or SQ), sublingual (SL), rectal (PR), vaginal, inhaled, oral (PO), or through the skin (topically). Each route of administration has some problems associated with it. It should be noted that interosseous and endotracheal are other routes of drug administration. However, elderly patients are not candidates for interosseous administration, and it is highly unlikely that the older adult will self-administer a drug endotracheally.

Obviously, the most direct route of administration of a drug into the bloodstream is by IV. IV administration places the medication directly into the circulation and en route to the tissues. In prehospital emergency care, many medications are administered via IV. However, it is unlikely that the geriatric patient will self-administer medications in this manner. Patients on chemotherapy or other IV therapy at home may administer these medications intravenously by devices known as a vascular access device (VAD) or venous access port (VAP). These terms are often used interchangeably.

A VAD is typically a catheter that is inserted into a peripheral or central vein for the purpose of administering antibiotics, chemotherapy, hydration, total parenteral nutrition (TPN), or for periodic sampling of blood. The hubs of these catheters are seen outside of the skin. Depending on the location of the device, it can remain in place for 30 to 360 days or longer. In contrast, a VAP consists of a plastic tube connected to a metal disc known as a port. The catheter and port are implanted under the skin, usually toward the upper end of the sternum with the catheter inserted into the subclavian vein. Access to the port is by inserting a needle through the skin and into the port.

VADs and VAPs are more commonly found in cancer patients receiving chemotherapy. Some of the anti-cancer drugs are very caustic to the veins and giving them by VAP reduces the incidence of damage to the vein. Common VADs and VAPs include dialysis devices used in patients with end-stage renal disease or heparin locks found in inserted into peripheral circulation.

Prehospital care providers assessing a patient with a VAD or VAP should be alert for complications of the devices. The complications of these devices are listed as follows.

Complications of Vascular Access Devices or Venous Access Ports

Bruising and swelling at the insertion site

Infection at the insertion site

Fever and chills

Swelling of the face or neck

Pain in the shoulders, arms, or neck

Complaint of difficulty injecting medications

Unless otherwise directed or permitted, prehospital care providers should not use VADs or VAPs for patient care.

KEY POINT

Some cancer patients may have a VAD or VAP to receive chemotherapy. These access routes should not be used in prehospital care unless absolutely necessary.

Intramuscular administration is another route of administration that gets the medication into the circulatory system at a relatively rapid rate. Like the IV administration of medications, the senior is not likely to self-medicate via IM injections, although there are a few chemotherapeutic or emergency drugs that can be self-administered by this route.

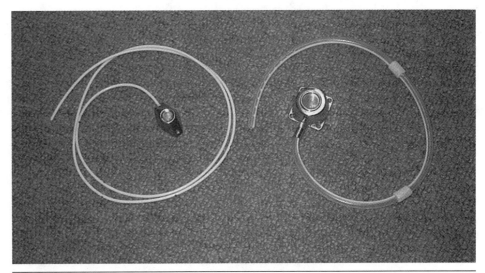

• FIGURE 7-1

Vascular access ports such as these are implanted into the upper arm (device on left) or upper chest (device on right). They allow for easier and less hazardous administration of chemotherapy. Paramedics will not access these ports during patient care.

Medications administered via IM injection are generally absorbed quickly. However, poor circulation to the injection site can slow absorption. Additionally, excess volumes of medication can cause the development of a sterile abscess. A sterile abscess prevents the absorption of the drug because the medication is walled off by the body's defenses and absorption is prevented. In most cases, the maximum amount of solution to be given IM should not exceed 3 ccs in the adult.

KEY POINT

Some patients self-medicate using IM injections in treating specific conditions. If too much solution is administered and it cannot be absorbed, a sterile abscess may form.

Some medications are administered by subcutaneous injection. For example, people with insulin-dependent diabetes will administer SC injections of insulin. Similar to IM injections, the rate of absorption is determined by the blood flow to the injection site. In the elderly, circulation to the skin and subcutaneous tissues may be reduced, slowing the absorption of the medication. Some medications are self-administered via this route. For example, Betaseron, which is used in the treatment of multiple sclerosis, and Infergen, which is used in the treatment of Hepatitis C, are self-administered subcutaneously.

KEY POINT

Some medications used to treat chronic conditions may be self-administered subcutaneously.

The sublingual route of administration provides for prompt absorption of a medication. Several cardiovascular medications, including nitroglycerin, are administered SL. Additionally, Procardia capsules used in treating hypertension can be crushed or emptied into the mouth to allow for SL absorption.

Some older adults may use suppositories to administer medications rectally. Commonly used suppositories include laxatives such as Ducolax. Another common PR medication is Compazine, which is used to treat nausea and vomiting. The rectum is highly vascular and the rate of absorption of a drug administered in this way is generally quick. However, absorption may be erratic depending on the contents and circulation of the rectum. Additionally, irritation of the rectum can occur with some drugs.

KEY POINT

Many suppositories are kept refrigerated. Look in the refrigerator when surveying the residence for medications the patient may use.

Inhaled medications are aerosol medications such as bronchodilators used in the treatment of asthma or chronic obstructive pulmonary disease. Drugs such as albuterol are self-administered through a metered-dose inhaler or by a nebulizer. A metered amount of medication or drug in mist form is inhaled into the lungs where it dilates the bronchi and bronchioles, allowing the patient to breathe easier.

Most of the medications used by the elderly are orally administered. Pills, capsules, tablets, and some liquid forms of medications are swallowed. Absorption is usually in the stomach or gastrointestinal tract. The rate of absorption of orally administered medications is slow. Some medications affect the acidity of the stomach and may not be absorbed entirely or may be partially destroyed by the acidity. Additionally, some medications can be affected by gastric contents. For example, the absorption of some antibiotics (tetracyclines) is prevented by dairy products or antacids.

Several medications are administered topically. With this type of administration, a drug is in an ointment or cream that is applied to the skin or the drug is contained in a patch that is attached to the skin. The medication is then continuously administered to the patient over a period of several hours. A nitroglycerin patch is an example of this route of administration. Other medications administered topically include corticosteroids and hormone replacement therapy. The rate of administration is affected by the circulation to the skin and, in the older adult, may be considerably delayed. When applying a drug to the skin, the skin must be intact to prevent rapid absorption into the body, which may cause adverse effects.

KEY POINT

Some patients self-administer medications such as nitroglycerin through the skin to ensure a gradual but continuous rate of administration.

The dosage of the medication will also affect its absorption rate. Higher dosages or higher concentrations of the medication will increase the absorption rate. In some cases, giving a loading dose of a medication quickly brings about a therapeutic effect, after which smaller, maintenance doses can be given to continue the therapeutic effect of the drug. Consider the prehospital administration of lidocaine in the treatment of premature ventricular contractions. An initial "loading" dose is given followed by a continuous flow by IV drip. The loading dose promptly brings the lidocaine to therapeutic levels and the slow IV drip maintains those levels.

The form of the drug will also affect its rate of absorption. Many oral medications are coated (enteric coating) to prevent quick breakdown in the stomach. This coating slows the drug's absorption. Other medications are formulated for sustained or prolonged release to maintain therapeutic levels over several hours or an entire day.

KEY POINT

Both route of administration and dose of the drug affect the absorption of the medication.

Once in the circulatory system, the drug needs to be transported to the target site. Many drugs pass from the blood vessels into the tissues without difficulty, thus taking effect quickly, however, these effects may be short-lived. Other drugs are attached to proteins or lipids (fats) in the blood that may enhance or delay their distribution to the tissues.

The status of the patient's circulatory system is a critical factor in drug distribution. If blood flow to the peripheral tissues is impaired, the drug will first circulate through the vital organs such as the heart, lungs, brain, liver, and kidneys before reaching the outlying areas.

KEY POINT

Blood flow to the area where a drug is given affects its rate of distribution. Giving an IM or SC injection into an area that has reduced blood flow will slow the drug's distribution.

When some drugs enter the circulatory system, parts of the dose attach to a protein (albumin) in the blood. The protein-bound drug becomes inactive and tends to form a drug reservoir. This reservoir is used to maintain the therapeutic action of the medication. There is an equal portion of the dose that is not attached to serum protein, and this is known as a free, or unbound, drug. As the free drug is used, transformed, metabolized, and excreted, the amount of free drug decreases. Since there must be an equal amount of bound and unbound medication, as the free drug is depleted, the protein-bound drug is released and therapeutic levels are continued.

The bound–unbound nature of some medications can adversely affect the older adult. Because of changes in the elderly patient's body water, fat, and muscle mass, drug distribution can be significantly affected. As a result, free medications may be more concentrated and have a more pronounced effect on the patient. The concentration of free drug is also a concern in patients who are taking multiple medications that compete for serum proteins. If two or more medications are seeking to bind with the same protein, the result is more free drug and an increased risk for toxic effects. Examples of medications that can compete for binding proteins include some oral hypoglycemic (antidiabetic) drugs and aspirin. Consider a person with adult-onset diabetes taking aspirin and an oral hypoglycemic medication (Dymelor, Glucotrol, Diabenese). Because of drug interactions and the competition for protein sites, a fatal hypoglycemic reaction may occur.

KEY POINT

The therapeutic effects of protein-bound drugs may last for long periods of time. Because there are always equal amounts of protein-bound and free drug, the drug can be slowly released to the tissues.

Protein-bound medications may take longer to metabolize, and their effects may be prolonged. Because the half-life of the drug is prolonged, the effects of the medication last considerably longer. For example, the effects of diazepam (Valium) are prolonged in the elderly. If the elderly patient were to follow the dosing schedule for a younger adult, they could suffer an overdose.

Metabolism and Excretion

Once inside the body's circulatory system, the drug is distributed throughout the body where it undergoes a change. This change, called biotransformation, occurs as the medication is converted from its initial state to a metabolite, making the drug less toxic to the tissues. The biotransformation, also called metabolism, primarily takes place in the liver, however, other organs such as the kidneys, lungs, and gastrointestinal system may also be involved.

The rate of metabolism of a drug will depend, in part, on the route of administration. Medications taken orally pass through the liver before making their way to the rest of the body. This "first-pass" metabolism reduces the amount of medication available to the body. To reduce the effects of first-pass metabolism, a higher dose of the medication can be given or the drug can be given by another route. For example, drugs given by injection (IV, SC, or IM) or drugs given as suppositories will avoid first-pass metabolism.

In the elderly or in those with impaired liver function, the metabolism of the medication can be delayed. In such patients, a drug could accumulate to toxic levels. For example, lidocaine is metabolized by the liver. Therefore, in heart attack victims over the age of 70 or in those with hepatic disease or congestive heart failure, the loading dose of lidocaine is cut in half.

KEY POINT

Drug metabolism in a patient with impaired liver function will be prolonged, therefore the effects of the drug will be longer lasting and the medication could accumulate to toxic levels.

It is also important to note that drug interactions can alter the rate of metabolism. In the liver, certain enzymes are responsible for the breakdown of medications in the bloodstream. Some drugs interfere with these enzymes, delaying biotransformation of the drugs and prolonging their effects. Not only can medications interfere with the metabolism of other drugs, beverages such as grapefruit juice also impede the enzyme responsible for metabolizing certain medications. Many older adults enjoy grapefruit juice in the morning. Unfortunately, this can prolong metabolism of many common drugs including (brand name shown in parentheses):

Alprazolam (Xanax)	Lidocaine
Astemizole (Hismanal)	Lovastatin (Mevacor)
Carbamazepine (Tegretol)	Midazolam (Versed)
Cisapride (Propulsid)	Nifedipine (Procardia)
Corticosteroids	Quinidine
Diazepam (Valium)	Simvastatin (Zocor)
Diltiazem (Cardizem)	Triazolam (Halcion)
Erythromycin	Terfenadine (Seldane)
Felodipine (Plendil)	Verapamil (Calan)

Once the drug has entered the body, it is eventually removed from the body through excretion. The primary organ that excretes the drug is the kidney, however, the gastrointestinal system, lungs, and skin can also excrete the drug and its metabolites.

The kidneys can excrete the drug's metabolites or the actual drug. Many drugs are excreted by the kidneys unchanged from their original form. With advancing age and decreased renal function, excretion of the drug through the kidneys is delayed. For those medications that are excreted unchanged, this prolongs the time the drug is in the system, thus prolonging the effects of the drug. Some medications are partially reabsorbed by the kidneys and returned to circulation.

Excretion of the drug can also occur in the intestines. After being metabolized by the liver, the metabolites are transported into the duodenum where they are excreted in the feces. As with the kidneys, some drugs are reabsorbed by the intestines and returned to circulation. Once back in the bloodstream, they are, if unchanged, metabolized by the liver or excreted by the kidneys.

The lungs excrete medications that are inhaled or those that consist of alcohols or other volatile substances. In the elderly patient, excretion by the lungs is affected by normal and pathological changes in the lungs such as the loss of alveoli or the loss of elasticity of the airways. A decrease in lung function can lengthen the time until the drug is excreted by the lungs.

The skin excretes drugs through sweating. This is an ineffective and minimal way of eliminating medications. Because of this, a patient may have an unusual body odor or some skin reaction to the excreted drug. In the elderly, a decreased number of sweat glands may inhibit excretion of medication through the skin.

FACTORS AFFECTING DRUG USE IN THE ELDERLY

There are several factors that complicate drug use in the senior population. The previous discussion focused on the basics of pharmokinetics (actions of drugs) on the patient. There are a number of other aspects that contribute to prescription drug problems in the older adult. Two of the bigger problems include the actual prescribing of the drug and patient compliance—making sure that the patient takes the medication and takes it correctly.

When requesting a prescription, a patient may be looking for a quick fix or responding to a recently aired television commercial. With the relaxation of direct-to-consumer rules regarding media commercials for medications, the pharmaceutical industry has been advertising drugs in various media—television, radio, and print. The result is an increased demand on the doctor for the advertised medication. With advertising telling the viewer to, "Ask your doctor about . . . ," 35 percent of patients over 65 years of age insist on trying the new medication. Frequently, doctors comply with the request.

KEY POINT

Direct-to-consumer advertising works! Seniors ask their doctors about and sometime receive drugs based on advertising hype. For those seniors with Internet access, information on health-related Web sites such as WebMD or Intelihealth could prompt the senior to ask for certain medications.

Because time constraints often limit the doctor's time with the patient, some doctors have written prescriptions to provide a quick fix. This is not to say that the doctors are totally responsible. Patients often expect a prescription at the end of their visit and feel disappointed if they don't get one.

Medication errors can occur if the medication schedule is too confusing. Dosing schedules can be hard to remember—Take one every four hours . . . Take one every three hours . . . Take one twice a day . . . Take two in the morning and one at bedtime. Pillboxes are available to help the senior remember the medications they need to take. Unfortunately, someone has to put the pills in the box for it to be of any benefit!

KEY POINT

Confusion over medication schedules can lead to medication errors. A pillbox can help reduce the risk of this type of error.

Occasionally, the patient will self-medicate without a doctor's advice. There may be medications leftover from a previous illness and, though a current condition may be different, the signs or symptoms may be similar. The

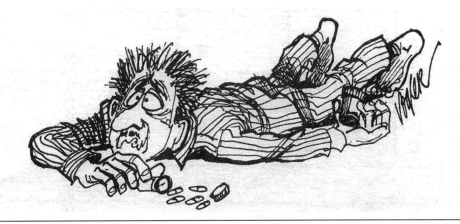

• FIGURE 7-2
Confusion over medication regimen could lead to serious consequences.
Source: Courtesy of EES Publications.

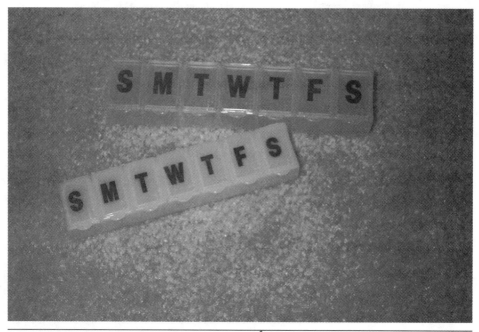

• FIGURE 7-3

Organizing medications can reduce or eliminate drug errors.

older adult will attempt to save money by taking the old medication, often to their detriment. Drug interactions can be fatal.

The prehospital care provider should suspect self-medication if they see a number of prescription drug bottles with varying dates of issue. When asking a patient about current medications, ask about prior medications. Look in the medicine cabinet for indications of self-medication.

Additionally, old medications may be expired. Recent evidence suggests that expired drugs retain their potency long after the expiration date. Other medications do change and either lose their effectiveness or become toxic.

Not only will the senior self-medicate with previously prescribed drugs, the senior may seek out a family member or neighbor and get medications from them to see if those drugs will alleviate their distress.

With the increasing availability of over-the-counter herbal remedies such as ginkgo biloba, ginseng, St. John's wort, and others, the patient may be tempted to try these remedies. Again, drug interactions can pose life-threatening effects. The prehospital care provider needs to ask the patient which over-the-counter medications or herbal remedies the patient has taken.

KEY POINT

Be alert for over-the-counter remedies, including herbal supplements.

There are a number of reasons that seniors may have difficulty complying with prescription medication guidelines. One major reason is that the senior may not understand how the medication should be taken or what the medication is expected to do, including any adverse effects. When a patient encounters an adverse effect that they were not expecting, the patient may call 9-1-1 for assistance. Estimates ranging from 10 to 20 percent of all hospital admissions are related to prescription drug side effects. "Essentials of Clinical Geriatrics," *American Family Physician,* vol 56, no. 7.

Other problems associated with compliance include: forgetting to take the drug; being confused about the drug regimen; inability to afford the medications; failure to complete the entire course of therapy; lack of motivation due to depression; not getting the desired results quickly; and problems with the container, including being unable to read the label.

With aging, people become forgetful. As was discussed in the chapter on dementia, patients with Alzheimer's disease become increasingly forgetful. Even without dementia, benign forgetfulness could cause a senior to skip a dose. Occasionally, a patient may forget that they took a dose, and then take a second dose. If the second dose is not remembered, a third dose may be taken. Under- or overmedication can be harmful or fatal.

With multiple drugs, the dosing regimen can be confusing. Sometimes the patient will remember to take the right amount of medication, whereas at other times they take too little. Again, patients can overdose or underdose, which results in physical distress and a call to 9-1-1.

Recently, the media has focused on the high cost of prescription drugs, at times citing examples of exorbitant costs. Patients who do not have adequate health insurance may not be able to afford their medications. If the drugs are unaffordable or out of the patient's price range, the older adult may go without taking the medication or take steps to afford some form of therapy. Older adults have been known to cut pills in half, reducing the dose; skip pills, saving some for later; use expired or stored medications; or not eat properly. There are cases where the older adult, faced with eating or taking medications to prolong life, has turned to eating pet food. The prehospital care provider needs to be aware of these factors when assessing the elderly and evaluating the older adult's ability to provide self-care.

KEY POINT

To save money, an older adult on a fixed income may skip the drug, skip meals, or cut pills in half. Doctors, pharmacies, and others suggest the cost of a prescription can be reduced by getting a double-sized dose and cutting the pills in half.

Older patients often like to save some of a prescription for a future onset of the same illness. This is especially true with antibiotics. For example, a patient with an upper respiratory infection feels better after a few days on the medication so they stop taking the drug, putting a few pills away for later. They are surprised when the infection returns.

If the patient is depressed, they may not be motivated to fill their prescriptions or, after getting the prescription filled, may not want to take the medications. As discussed in the chapter on psychosocial changes, there is an increased risk for suicide in the elderly. The prehospital care provider needs to be alert for the hoarding of sedative drugs that could be used later in a suicide attempt.

In this society, we have become accustomed to the quick fix. The media advertises fast food, in-and-out dry cleaning, and prompt resolution of whatever ails a person. One commercial years ago advertised, "When you haven't got time for the pain . . ." In anticipation of a quick fix to an ailment, the patient can become frustrated with the slow progress in treating the disorder and stop taking

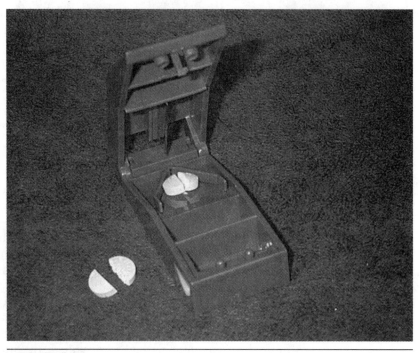

• FIGURE 7-4
Using a pill splitter can help reduce cost of medications for older adults on a limited income.

the medication. One older adult who called EMS complained of a urinary tract infection for which she had been prescribed an antibiotic. She was upset when, after taking one pill, the infection and pain were still present. She felt the antibiotic was useless.

Safety in the storage and handling of medications is important. When young children are present, childproof pill containers are important. When the only people near or around the medication are adults, child-resistant caps on the containers are unnecessary and can pose a problem to the older adult. Some seniors with arthritis cannot open the pill bottles and are therefore unable to take their medication. Not only are the containers childproof, they are also elderly proof.

Some older adults are at a greater risk for medication errors than others. When the prehospital care provider arrives at the scene, they should consider several factors that could increase the risk of a drug error. These include:

- Living alone or isolated from others.
- No family doctor or a history of "doctor shopping." Look for multiple medications from different doctors.
- Dementia or forgetfulness.
- Depression or lack of motivation to care for themselves.
- Alcohol or drug abuse.
- No insurance or lack of monetary support.
- English as a second language. Foreign patients who do not speak the same language as their doctor are more apt to be confused about the medication they are taking.
- Expecting a quick cure or fast relief from symptoms.

This next section will address certain medications that can create problems for the older adult. These problems include side effects, contraindications, and drug interactions. The prehospital care provider can often spot a potential problem with a medication as the provider can see first-hand what medications the patient is taking. Being familiar with the medications that could create a problem in the elderly gives the prehospital care provider the opportunity to alert the emergency department physician before a drug interaction or side effect becomes life threatening.

Before discussing specific prescription medications that may cause a problem in the elderly, it is important to consider over-the-counter medications that may interact with other medications. Nonprescription drugs are popular. Millions of dollars are spent annually for over-the-counter remedies. There are several general types of medications that may cause problems. These include nonsteroidal anti-inflammatory drugs (NSAIDs), antihistamines or decongestants, laxatives, and antacids.

NSAIDs including all nonprescription pain relievers such as aspirin, ibuprofen, and naproxen sodium. Use of these drugs increases the risk for many different problems.

Aspirin is associated with an increased risk of gastrointestinal bleeding and ulcers. Patients on anticoagulants such as Coumadin have a significant risk of bleeding, and that risk is increased by aspirin. Patients on medications that could affect sight may have an increased risk of diminished vision. Aspirin in high doses can reduce a person's hearing. Other NSAIDs also increase the risk of gastrointestinal bleeding, and, along with aspirin, may also increase the risk of bruising.

Antihistamines and other decongestants also pose risks for the elderly. Some nondrowsy formulas can increase a person's blood pressure to dangerously high levels. They can cause confusion, blurred vision, and an increase in intraocular pressure (glaucoma). Antihistamines may cause constipation as well as urinary retention, which, in turn, can lead to delirium.

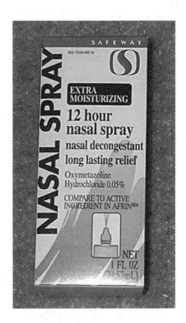

• FIGURE 7-5
Some nasal sprays are vaso-constrictors and can elevate blood pressure.

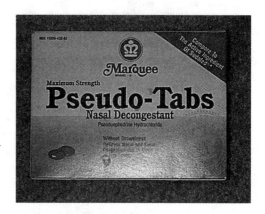

• FIGURE 7-6
Decongestants with pseudo-
ephedrine will elevate blood
pressure.

The older adult frequently abuses laxatives. Excessive use of laxatives can alter electrolytes, cause dehydration, and interfere with the effectiveness of other drugs.

Many antacids contain large quantities of sodium, posing a danger to those patients who need to restrict sodium intake. Water retention is associated with increased sodium, which could worsen congestive heart failure.

> ### KEY POINT
>
> Over-the-counter medications are not benign. Watch out for excessive use of NSAIDs, antihistamines, laxatives, and antacids.

Specific Prescription Medications

There are a large number of medications that elderly patients should use with caution. Although many of these drugs may not be contraindicated in the senior population, their use can cause problems that might result in a call to EMS. These drugs are initially discussed by type of medication along with specific names, actions, and adverse effects. The astute prehospital care provider can identify complications associated with prescription drug use and alert the emer-

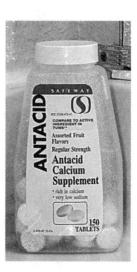

• FIGURE 7-7
Many antacids may contain
sodium.

gency department physician. The types of medications that may cause problems in the elderly patient include:

- **Antianxiety medications.** Medications that alleviate anxiety or panic and tranquilize the patient.
- **Antidepressants.** Medications that alleviate depression.
- **Antinausea and gastrointestinal medications.** Medications used to treat nausea/vomiting and ulcers.
- **Arthritis drugs.** Medications that alleviate the pain of arthritis.
- **Cardiovascular medications.** Medications used to treat cardiac dysrhythmias and hypertension.
- **Oral hypoglycemic drugs.** Medications that reduce high blood sugar in the diabetic.
- **Muscle relaxants.** Medications that relieve spasms and help in rehabilitation.
- **Pain relievers.** Medications that alleviate pain and discomfort.

Antianxiety. Antianxiety medications include the class of drugs known as benzodiazepines. The more commonly prescribed benzodiazepines include (brand name shown in parentheses):

Alprazolam (Xanax)	Chlordiazepoxide (Librium)
Clonazepam (Klonopin)	Clorazepate dipotassium (Tranxene)
Diazepam (Valium)	Flurazepam (Dalmane)
Lorazepam (Ativan)	Oxazepam (Serax)
Temazepam (Restoril),	

The actions of these drugs relieve anxiety, relax skeletal muscles, act as anticonvulsants, and produce sedation. These medications are prescribed based on their onset and duration of action. Clonazepam, clorazepate, diazepam, and flurazepam have longer durations than their counterparts. Clorazepate, diazepam, and flurazepam have a quick onset of actions.

Of the benzodiazepines, diazepam and alprazolam need to be mentioned as posing specific hazards in the elderly. Diazepam has a long half-life ranging from 14 to 100 hours. The half-life of the medication can be equated with the age of the patient. In the elderly, the drug has a greater volume of distribution throughout the body. Diazepam is metabolized in the liver; however, its metabolites are active, meaning that they continue to prolong the effects of the medication. For example, one of the metabolites of diazepam is tamazepam, which metabolizes to another active chemical, oxazepam. Elderly patients on diazepam may exhibit prolonged drowsiness, ataxia, dizziness, and weakness.

Alprazolam is another antianxiety medication that needs to be discussed as a medication with potential problems for the elderly. Alprazolam is a short-acting benzodiazepine with a fast onset used in the treatment of anxiety and panic attacks. Alprazolam has a high potential for addiction, thus regular, long-term use of this medication has not been recommended. The side effects of alprazolam are the same as with diazepam. Because of the adverse effects of these antianxiety medications, the older adult has an increased chance of falling and sustaining soft tissue injuries and fractures.

Drug interactions with benzodiazepines may also occur. Patients taking digitalis preparations are at an increased risk for digitalis toxicity. Patients with Parkinson's disease taking levodopa may notice a decreased effect of the levodopa. The elderly patient who abuses alcohol is at substantial risk for adverse effects from benzodiazepines as alcohol potentiates the effects of the drugs.

Antidepressants. Antidepressants are frequently prescribed to help a person overcome clinical depression. There are several different types of antidepressants, including tricyclics, selective serotonin reuptake inhibitors (SSRI), and monoamine oxidase (MAO) inhibitors.

Tricyclic antidepressants include the generic amitriptyline (brand names: Elavil, Endep, Etrafon, Limbitrol, Sinequan, and Triavil). These drugs, although effective in treating depression, have also been prescribed for urinary incontinence. Use of these medications may lead to urinary retention, dizziness, and drowsiness. Additional adverse effects include dry mouth, blurred vision, and constipation. As mentioned earlier, urinary retention and fecal impaction have been known to cause delirium in the elderly.

One tricyclic antidepressant to note is doxepin (Sinequan). Sinequan is often used to treat depression when sedating the patient is a desirable effect. Side effects of doxepin include hypotension, sedation, confusion, dizziness, constipation, dry mouth, and weight gain.

Other antidepressants include the class of medications known as SSRIs. This class of medications includes drugs such as venlafaxine (Effexor), paroxetene (Paxil), fluoxetine (Prozac), and sertraline (Zoloft). Of these medications, paroxetene is considered the most powerful sedative. Using this medication can increase the chance of falling and sustaining injuries. Other than sedation, the side effects of paroxetene include hypotension, tachycardia, headache, nervousness, insomnia, dry mouth, and pain in the ears and eyes. Using this drug with alcohol will increase its effect or lead to toxicity.

MAO inhibitors are also used to treat depression. Although not prescribed as often as in the past, many elderly take an MAO inhibitor to treat depression. The two MAO inhibitors commonly prescribed are phenylzine (Nardil) and tranylcypromine (Parnate). MAO affects the metabolism of neurotransmitters such as epinephrine and norepinephrine. If MAO is blocked, the levels of these neurotransmitters and others are increased, producing an antidepressant effect. Although these drugs have shown a high degree of effectiveness, they pose problems in the elderly. MAO inhibitors should not be used in patients with hypertension, cardiovascular or cerebrovascular disease, heart failure, or reduced liver or kidney function. Use of MAO inhibitors may increase the depressant effects of alcohol and oral antidiabetic medications. Patients on MAO inhibitors may experience a hypertensive crisis and a variety of cardiac dysrhythmias.

Of particular note, in calls where advanced cardiac life support is necessary, the prehospital care provider should exercise extreme caution when giving the patient any catecholamine (epinephrine, dopamine, etc.). Because of the nature of MAO inhibitors, the effects of these prehospital drugs can be significantly increased. For example, if a patient takes an MAO inhibitor and the paramedic needs to administer dopamine, the paramedic should be prepared to administer 10 percent of the normal dose. A dopamine infusion at a higher dose can precipitate hypertensive crisis or other adverse effects. If in doubt, contact medical control for complete instructions for on-scene care of the critically ill patient who is taking an MAO inhibitor.

Antinausea and other gastrointestinal medications.   Patients on chemotherapy or those with gastric upset may take medications that reduce nausea and vomiting. One such medication is trimethobenzamide (Tigan). This medication can be given orally or by rectal suppository, but it should be used with extreme caution in the elderly. Severe adverse reactions can occur in patients over the age of 60 years. These reactions include confusion, disorientation, agitation, and psychotic-like symptoms. Other side effects include drowsiness, blurred vision, dizziness, headache, and muscle cramps. Seizures and depression are possible, but rare.

Gastrointestinal problems that can also occur in the elderly involve excess acidity resulting in gastroesophageal reflux disorder (GERD). GERD is described as a burning sensation in the esophagus and upper chest and throat and is caused by stomach acids entering the esophagus. Patients with GERD may be prescribed cimetidine (Tagamet). Cimetidine is also used in the treatment of gastric and duodenal ulcers. The drug works by inhibiting gastric acid secretion in the gastrointestinal system. The adverse effects of cimetidine include headache, dizziness, drowsiness, confusion, disorientation, psychosis, and hallucinations. Patients over 50 years of age have a higher risk of confusion than younger adults. Other drugs in this same class such as ranitidine (Zantac) and famotidine (Pepcid) are better tolerated by the elderly.

Arthritis medications.   Arthritis affects millions of older adults. People throughout the United States spend billions of dollars each year on over-the-counter and prescription pain relievers to alleviate the pain of arthritis. One prescription medication that should be used with caution in the elderly is indomethacin (Indocin). Indomethacin belongs in the class of drugs known as NSAIDs. Although all NSAIDs cause gastrointestinal irritation and ulcers along with gastric bleeding, indomethacin has a significantly higher rate of these side effects than other NSAIDs. Indomethacin has also been shown to worsen depression as well as aggravate Parkinson's disease and epilepsy. Other adverse effects of indomethacin include fluid retention, edema, dizziness, headache, and indigestion. Occasionally, the patient may complain of tinnitus.

Cardiovascular medications.   Many older adults take medications that affect the heart or lower blood pressure. There are eight medications that prehospital care providers should be aware of that may cause problems in the geriatric patient. Some of these medications are antidysrhythmics, whereas others are used to treat hypertension.

The antidysrhythmia medications include:

Amiodarone (Cordarone)
Digoxin (Lanoxin)
Disopyramide (Norpace)
Flecainide (Tambocor)
Verapamil (Calan, Isoptin)

Amiodarone is prescribed to treat ventricular and supraventricular dysrhythmias when other forms of treatment have not been successful. There has been recent controversy surrounding the use of amiodarone in pulseless ventricular tachycardia or ventricular fibrillation as indicated in the American Heart Association algorithms. At its May 5, 2001 meeting, the American Academy of Emergency Medicine Board of Directors adopted an official position statement, that stated,

> It is the position of the American Academy of Emergency Medicine that the use of amiodarone in refractory pulseless ventricular tachycardia or ventricular fibrillation (VT/VF) should not be considered the current "standard of care" for this condition. The Academy does not condemn nonresearch use of amiodarone given the absence of any proven beneficial alternatives, however, there is currently no reason to conclude that its use is mandatory or represents a "standard of care." Until ongoing or future research clarifies this issue, emergency physicians should use their own discretion regarding antidysrhythmic therapy in patients with cardiac arrest.

With time and additional studies, the controversy over the use of amiodarone should wind down.

Amiodarone has a prolonged half-life, and older adults have an increased risk of toxicity because of its longer actions. Most elderly patients taking this drug experience some adverse effects that may include heart failure; hypotension; tachycardia; dizziness; fatigue; insomnia; bluish-gray tint to the skin of the face, arms, and neck; vomiting; blurred vision; and muscular incoordination. Patients using other medications such as digitalis, procainamide, warfarin, or other cardiac medications in conjunction with amiodarone may experience increased and perhaps toxic effects from these other drugs. Bradycardia has been known to occur in patients taking amiodarone and digitalis or calcium channel blockers (i.e., verapamil).

Digoxin is a digitalis preparation that is used to treat atrial fibrillation and, occasionally, congestive heart failure. The side effects of digoxin include other cardiac dysrhythmias such as heart blocks, drowsiness, fatigue, headache, vomiting, weakness, and blurred vision. One symptom of digitalis toxicity is a yellow tint to the vision.

Disopyramide is used to treat premature ventricular contractions and may be used in the treatment of supraventricular tachycardia. It tends to slow the heart rate. In the elderly, disopyramide may worsen congestive heart failure. Side effects of this medication include dry mouth, eyes, nose, and throat, difficulty urinating, headache, dizziness, blurred vision, and constipation. Although rare, hypotension, edema, dyspnea, and fainting have been reported.

Flecainide is used to treat potentially life-threatening ventricular heart rhythms, as well as a rhythm known as paroxysmal supraventricular tachycardia. Unfortunately, flecainide has serious side effects, including worsening congestive heart failure, chest pain, dyspnea, visual disturbances, dizziness, fatigue, abdominal pain, dry mouth, and blurred vision. These adverse reactions may outweigh the drug's usefulness in the elderly patient. Patients using flecainide may call 9-1-1 for assistance should they develop heart failure, chest pain, or experience palpitations.

Verapamil is used for a variety of cardiovascular conditions including angina and supraventricular rhythms, including atrial fibrillation, and in the treatment of high blood pressure. Side effects of verapamil include constipation, dizziness, lightheadedness, headache, loss of sensation, swelling of the hands/wrists and ankles/feet, hypotension, and bradycardia. If the patient becomes toxic, they may develop extreme hypotension, bradycardia, or congestive heart failure, and may experience cardiac dysrhythmias, including heart block and asystole. A number of medications adversely interact with verapamil and could worsen the patient's condition.

Antihypertensive drugs can pose problems in the elderly. The drugs include

Methyldopa (Aldoril, Aldomet)
Propranolol (Inderal)
Reserpine (Hydropres, Serpasil)

Of the three antihypertensive medications listed, both methyldopa and reserpine have a similar mode of action—they dilate the arteries in order to decrease the patient's blood pressure. Neither of these medications is used as a first-line treatment against hypertension, but may be found later in the treatment regimen. There are serious adverse side effects for each medication. The side effects for methyldopa include edema, dizziness, weakness, nasal congestion, and physical and mental slowing. It has also been known to cause sedation. The side effects of reserpine include severe depression, which may lead to suicide, weight gain, sedation, and tremors. Additional adverse side effects of reserpine are the same as those seen in methyldopa. Some studies have found reserpine to be safe and effective for use by elderly patients, whereas others have advocated against its use.

Propranolol uses a different mechanism to lower the patient's blood pressure—it lowers the heart rate and force of contraction. Although some studies have shown propranolol to be safe and effective for lowering blood pressure in the elderly, some patients report physical and mental slowing. It also has a long duration of action and may lead to severe hypotension in the older adult. Propranolol may cause fatigue, sleepiness, and depression. This drug should not be used in patients with underlying congestive heart failure, COPD, or asthma, as it could worsen each of these conditions.

KEY POINT

Cardiovascular medications are frequently prescribed as treatment for a variety of cardiovascular ailments. Although the intent of these medications is good, there are some drugs that can adversely impact the patient's quality of life.

Oral hypoglycemic drugs. Millions of older adults have been diagnosed with adult-onset diabetes mellitus. Initially, many are treated with diet and exercise. If they fail to control their blood sugar levels, they may be placed on an oral hypoglycemic medication. Two of these medications can pose problems for the elderly. These medications are chlorpropamide (Diabenese) and metformin (Glucophage).

Chlorpropamide is a long-acting, protein-bound medication that stimulates the pancreas to release more insulin. Since it is long-acting and because it is excreted by the kidneys, chlorpropamide is not recommended for use in the older patient with decreased kidney function. The prolonged action of this drug has been known to cause severe and occasionally fatal hypoglycemia. Diabetic patients who are not familiar with the signs and symptoms of hypoglycemia could succumb to the disorder before they know to call for help.

Metformin is a medication that acts by decreasing glucose production in the liver, as opposed to stimulating the release of insulin from the pancreas. This drug has also been known to be used simultaneously with insulin-releasing drugs. Of particular note and of significant danger in the elderly is the uncommon but potentially fatal side effect known as lactic acidosis. The signs and symptoms of lactic acidosis include hyperventilation, various muscle aches, fatigue, and sleepiness. The condition can progress to shock and acute heart failure. Older adults with decreased liver or kidney function should not use metformin.

KEY POINT

Monitor a patient's blood sugar as a routine component of patient assessment. Profound hypoglycemia in the elderly patient could be due to an oral hypoglycemic drug.

Muscle relaxants.   Muscle relaxants include those medications used to treat muscle spasms or other skeletal muscle pain. Two skeletal muscle relaxants that should be used with caution or avoided by the elderly include cyclobenzaprine (Flexeril) and methocarbamol (Robaxin). Although the exact mechanisms of their actions are unclear, the drugs are known to be central nervous system depressants. Typical adverse side effects include dizziness, drowsiness, blurred vision, and headache. Because of their CNS depressant activity, use of this drug may cause the elderly to fall and sustain soft tissue injuries and fractures.

Pain relievers.   Many older adults suffer from chronic pain caused by any number of conditions, including arthritis, cancer, fractures, muscle spasms, osteoporosis, or other disease. These seniors will often take multiple pain medications, including over-the-counter NSAIDs and prescription analgesics. There are four pain relief medications that could cause problems in a senior citizen. These medications include meperidine (Demerol), orphenadrine (Norflex, Norgesic), pentazocine (Talwin), and propoxyphene (Darvon, Darvocet).

Meperidine has been around for a number of years and has been known to be an effective narcotic analgesic. However, in the elderly, this drug can cause serious adverse side effects. Generally, the side effects of narcotic pain medications include drowsiness, nausea, vomiting, constipation, slowing of rate and depth of breathing, and hypotension. In the elderly, though, the drug's metabolite, normeperidine, can induce tremors or seizures. Additionally, meperidine can increase the effects or toxicity of other medications, including antidepressants or CNS depressants. Patients taking MAO inhibitors, SSRI drugs, and tricyclic antidepressants should avoid meperidine.

Orphenadrine is a non-narcotic pain reliever that is often combined with caffeine in a tablet form. The drug is used to treat skeletal muscle pain, but it does not act directly to relax tense skeletal muscles. Instead, it may have an analgesic effect or atropine-like action on the muscles. Orphenadrine has been known to cause lightheadedness, dizziness, and fainting. The injectable form of the drug contains sodium bisulfite, which has been known to cause severe allergy-like reactions. Other adverse effects of orphenadrine include tachycardia, palpitation, urinary retention, constipation, blurred vision, and drowsiness among many other reported effects.

Pentazocine is a narcotic analgesic that is as effective as codeine on a milligram-per-milligram basis. As with any narcotic, hypotension, dizziness, sleepiness, and respiratory depression are common side effects. Lightheadedness, disorientation, and fainting have been reported, as have urinary spasms, blurred vision, and ringing in the ears. Pentazocine's effects may be increased in patients with reduced liver or kidney function.

Propoxyphene has been frequently prescribed for pain management, although some critics claim that its effectiveness is not much better than aspirin. It is a narcotic analgesic and, in addition to the side effects seen with narcotic use, it has been known to cause seizures and irregular heart rhythms in the elderly. Propoxyphene is highly addictive and has been used by depressed patients to commit suicide. Adverse effects include lightheadedness, headache, weakness, elevated or depressed mood, hallucinations, and visual disturbances.

> ### KEY POINT
>
> Muscle relaxers and pain relievers are excellent tools in patient care, but they are potentially harmful when an older adult takes the drug in normal, therapeutic doses.

DRUGS THAT INTERFERE WITH HEARING

As indicated in the previous discussion, there are a number of drugs that have blurred vision as one of the adverse effects. Blurred vision cannot only impair the older adult's ability to provide self-care, it could lead to falls and other injuries or medication errors. However, many medications can also affect a person's hearing. One common adverse effect of some drugs is tinnitus, defined as a noise in the ears. The noise can consist of ringing, buzzing, or roaring that can be so loud that people other than the patient can hear it. Tinnitus can be an initial symptom caused by drugs that are considered ototoxic or harmful to a person's hearing.

Tinnitus that is severe and prolonged can interfere with a person's activities of daily living, including getting adequate rest. It can also interfere with hearing a doctor's instructions and with patient assessment. If the patient complains of a persistent noise, they may not hear or understand the questions the prehospital care provider asks. The list of medications that follows consists of many drugs that have been identified as having a potential for tinnitus. The list is available from and distributed by the American Tinnitus Association. The drugs are listed in alphabetical order and by brand or commonly known name.

Acromycin	Atrofen	Corgard
Actifed	Bactrim	Daypro
Adalat CC	Benadryl	Deconamine
Anatranil	BuSpar	Diamox
Anaprox	Capastat sulfate	Dilacor XR
Anestacon	Claritin	Disalcid
Asacol	Clinoril	Dolobid

Dyclone	Lopressor	Quinidex
Effexor	Lotensin	Rifater
Elavil	Medlomen	Rythmol
Eldepryl	Minipress	Salflex
Erythromycin	Mintezol	Septra
Equagesic	Moduretic	Sinequan
Eskalith	Nalfon	Stadol
Fansidar	Naprosyn	Streptomycin sulfate
Flexeril	Nebcin	Surmontil
Foscavir	Netromycin	Tambocor
Gantanol	Nipride	Tegretol
Gantrism	Norpramin	Temaril
Garamycin	Ornade	Ticlid
Hyperstat	Orudis	Timoptic
Hytrin	Oruvail	Tobramycin
Ilosone	Pamelor	Tolectin
Imdur	Parnate	Torecan
Indocin	Paxil	Triavil
Kerione	Periactin	Trilisate
Lariam	Phenergan	Vascor
Lasix	Plendil	Vasotec
Legratin	Prilosec	Wellbutrin
Lincocin	Prinivil	Xanax
Lithane	Procardia	Zestril
Lithium carbonate	Proventil	Ziac
Lodine	Prozac	Zoloft

KEY POINT

A patient may refuse to take a medication that interferes with their hearing.

A WORD ABOUT HERBAL SUPPLEMENTS

Many adults have begun using herbal supplements to enhance their health. With direct-to-consumer advertising hyping the effects of herbal supplements, many people have opted to try them as opposed to or in conjunction with prescription medications. Of the several hundred herbal remedies available, there are a few that are becoming increasingly popular with older adults. These over-the-counter supplements include St. John's wort, ginkgo biloba, garlic, ginger, ginseng, melatonin, valerian, and yohimbe.

St. John's wort has been used for centuries as an effective antidepressant as well as an effective treatment for burns, ulcers, and insect bites. It was first introduced as an antidepressant in the 1970s, but after articles appeared in the *British Medical Journal* in August 1996, the remedy's popularity increased tremendously. Although the exact mechanism of action is still not clearly understood, several theories have suggested a variety of actions. Some studies indicate that the herb acts like an MAO inhibitor, whereas others have suggested the herb works like an SSRI.

Side effects of St. John's wort include increased sensitivity to sunlight and gastrointestinal upset. Of particular note is that the herb may interfere with other drugs such as heart medications, antidepressants, and antiseizure drugs. A recent study by the National Institute of Health found that St. John's wort decreases the blood levels and effectiveness of HIV drugs such as Indinavir and other antiretrovial agents. Otherwise, St. John's wort, when used in average amounts, has been found to be relatively safe.

Ginkgo biloba, another popular herbal remedy, has also been around for centuries. The mechanism of action for ginkgo is in the inhibition of the body's platelet activation factor, a substance that is involved in many biological processes, including asthma, blood flow, and the formation of blood clots. Thus, ginkgo has been used in the treatment of stroke, heart attack, decreased memory, impotence, macular degeneration, ringing in the ears, asthma, and more. Because platelet activation factor plays a key role in the formation of blood clots, older adults who have bleeding disorders should avoid ginkgo. Prehospital control of bleeding may be more difficult in patients taking this supplement. Some people have complained of irritability, nausea, vomiting, diarrhea, and restlessness. In a normal dose, however, side effects from gingko biloba are minimal.

Garlic has been touted as having multiple benefits, including reducing cholesterol, lowering blood pressure, blocking blood clot formation, and fighting against viral or bacterial infections. Most of the time there are only minimal adverse effects with garlic consumption such as an offensive odor, heartburn, and gas. However, a patient may experience prolonged bleeding with the use of garlic. Garlic should be used with caution by people with bleeding disorders or those taking anticoagulants.

Ginger is often used as a spice, however, it has also been used to relieve nausea, especially in people prone to motion sickness. It has been advocated as an anti-inflammatory supplement to treat arthritis. It also tends to block or delay blood clotting. Like garlic and other herbal supplements, the adverse effects are minimal when taken in the suggested amounts. However, large doses have been known to cause CNS depression and abnormal cardiac rhythms.

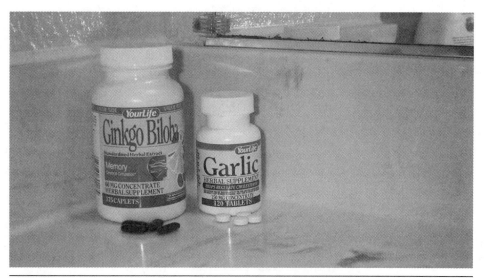

• FIGURE 7-8

Look for herbal supplements that could interfere with prescribed medications.

The literature on herbal supplements suggests that ginseng can be used to boost energy and sexual stamina and decrease the effects of aging. Side effects of ginseng include breast tenderness, nervousness, headache, hypertension, and abnormal vaginal bleeding. Diabetics may experience hypoglycemia, especially if they are using insulin. Blood clotting may be delayed and bleeding times prolonged in patients who take ginseng on a regular basis.

Marijuana, although not an herbal supplement, is occasionally used by cancer patients to ameliorate the nausea and vomiting associated with chemotherapy. It is also used by cancer patients to overcome the anorexia caused by the cancer-fighting drugs. Many states have approved laws allowing the sale and distribution of marijuana for medical use. In May 2001, the U.S. Supreme Court declared that Congress' law banning the sale or distribution of marijuana was clear, and that marijuana was not medically beneficial. In spite of this setback, cancer patients are continuing to smoke marijuana to enhance their quality of life. The active ingredient in marijuana, tetrahydracannabinol (THC), is said to provide relief of nausea and vomiting while stimulating the patient's appetite. Other than relieving nausea, vomiting, and anorexia, THC causes euphoria, sleepiness, altered perceptions, and hallucinations in high doses. Some people experience paranoia when using the drug.

KEY POINT

Some states have legalized the use of medical marijuana in treatment of nausea, vomiting, and anorexia from chemotherapy.

Melatonin is a hormone produced by the pineal gland located at the base of the brain. It regulates sleep cycles and the hormonal changes that trigger sexual maturity. It has been promoted as a treatment for jet lag and other forms of insomnia. Since melatonin can affect the biological clock, it has been suggested for depression, particularly seasonal affective disorder (SAD). Melatonin has also been touted in the treatment of cancer, as it also affects the immune system.

Side effects of melatonin include confusion, drowsiness, sleepwalking, and disorientation. The older adult may have an increased chance of falls and injuries caused by the adverse effects of melatonin. Melatonin is contraindicated in patients with a history of stroke, depression, or liver or kidney disease. If the patient may be a candidate for surgery, let the emergency department know of the patient's melatonin use.

Valerian has been used as a sedative for many years. Research indicates that it improves the quality of sleep. It is also used to treat restlessness and nervousness. Adverse effects of valerian include palpitations, upset stomach, headache, excitability, and uneasiness. Blurred vision and morning grogginess have also been reported. Although no drug interactions have been reported, valerian should not be used by people taking CNS depressants or tranquilizers.

Yohimbe has been described as a male aphrodisiac and is used to treat impotence, erectile dysfunction, and postural hypotension. Side effects of yohimbe include dizziness, insomnia, anxiety, hypertension, and tachycardia. Large doses of yohimbe may cause hallucinations, weakness, and paralysis. Yohimbe may decrease the effectiveness of antidepressants and drugs used to treat high blood pressure.

Herb	Uses	Adverse Effects	Interactions
St. John's wort	Antidepressant Wound care	Increased sensitivity to sunlight Gastrointestinal upset	May interfere with antiretroviral drugs
Ginkgo biloba	Stroke Heart attack Poor memory Impotence Macular degeneration Tinnitus	Increased bleeding Irritability Nausea/vomiting Diarrhea Restlessness	Increases effects of anticoagulant drugs.
Garlic	Lower cholesterol Lower blood pressure Anticoagulant Antibiotic/antiviral	Garlic odor Heartburn Gas	Use with caution in patients with bleeding disorders or those who use anticoagulants
Ginger	Relieve nausea Arthritis	Large dose can cause CNS depression and dysrhythmias	Use with caution in patients who use anticoagulants
Ginseng	Boost energy Increase sexual stamina Reduce effects of aging	Nervousness Headache Hypertension Hypoglycemia	
Melatonin	Insomnia Glaucoma	Grogginess Drowsiness Sleepwalking Disorientation	May increase effects of other tranquilizers. Do not take with zinc or magnesium.
Valerian	Sedation Improve sleep Restlessness Nervousness	Palpitations Upset stomach Headache Irritability Blurred vision Morning grogginess	Avoid when taking CNS depressants such as tranquilizers
Yohimbe	Impotence Erectile dysfunction	Dizziness Insomnia Anxiety Hypertension Tachycardia Hallucinations Weakness/Paralysis	Decrease effectiveness of antidepressants and antihypertensive drugs

KEY POINT

The herbal supplement industry is huge. Many people use supplements daily. When asking about a patient's medication use, be sure to include questions about herbal supplements.

SUMMARY

This chapter discussed aspects of pharmacology with particular attention to the elderly patient. Initially, the chapter presented information about drug names and forms. It also discussed drug absorption and distribution, as well as drug metabolism and excretion. After establishing or reviewing some of the basics of pharmacology, the chapter discussed factors affecting drug use and compliance by older adults. Seniors have a multitude of factors that can affect the safe and effective use of prescribed drugs.

Next, the chapter presented the hazards of specific classes of medications, from antianxiety medications to pain relievers. Since the older adult may have a multitude of drugs in their medicine cabinet, the prehospital care provider needs to be aware of drugs that can pose specific problems in the elderly. Not only do these medications pose their own risks, they can also interact with other drugs, increasing the risk of a serious, and perhaps lethal, adverse reaction.

This chapter also presented a list of medications that can interfere with a patient's hearing. Tinnitus, or a ringing, buzzing, or roaring in the ears, can affect the older adult's quality of life and interfere with the activities of daily living. Tinnitus can also affect interpersonal communications and hamper patient assessment during a critical emergency.

Finally, the chapter discussed a few of the herbal supplements that seniors may take to self-treat certain conditions. Although most of these herbal remedies have minimal adverse effects, they can interfere with other medications.

Armed with this information, the prehospital care provider can recognize potential problems with drugs the older adult may be taking. The prehospital care provider can then alert the emergency department physician of their findings at the scene of the emergency, possibly enhancing overall patient care.

ON THE JOB

Upon arriving at the scene, you are escorted to the patient by the patient's wife, a woman who appears to be in her 60s. She tells you that her husband has not been feeling well, "He's had that nasty flu that's been going around. Now he seems worse." On reaching the patient, you find a 69-year-old man complaining that he has had a severe headache that "will not go away." He adds that along with the flu, nasal congestion, and cough, the headache has just gotten worse. On assessing the patient, you note that his vital signs are blood pressure at 210/120, pulse 98 and regular, and breathing noisy at 22 per minute. As you are gathering information about his condition, you notice several over-the-counter medications on his nightstand. These include, Sudafed, Afrin, and aspirin. In the man's bathroom, you also find yohimbe, ginkgo biloba, garlic tablets, and hydrochlorothiazide. Why is the man's blood pressure abnormally high? Is the man suffering a stroke? How do the medications the man is taking affect his overall well-being?

8

Medical Emergencies: Common Problems Seen in the Elderly

OBJECTIVES

At the end of the chapter, the reader will be able to:

1 List the signs, symptoms, and treatment of patients with dyspnea from COPD.
2 List the signs, symptoms, and treatment of acute respiratory failure.
3 Discuss deep vein thrombosis and its role in the development of pulmonary embolism.
4 List the signs, symptoms, and treatment of pulmonary embolism.
5 List the signs, symptoms, and treatment of bacterial pneumonia.
6 Determine a normal blood pressure for an adult of a certain age using the standard guideline.
7 State the systolic and diastolic blood pressures that indicate hypertension.
8 Given a list of medications, identify those medications that are used to treat hypertension.
9 Describe the treatment for a patient with hypertensive crisis and hypertensive encephalopathy.
10 List the signs, symptoms, and treatment for left ventricular failure with pulmonary edema.
11 List the signs, symptoms, and treatment for a dissecting aortic aneurysm.
12 Identify and treat a patient whose pacemaker has failed to capture.
13 List the signs, symptoms, and treatment for stroke and TIA.
14 List 13 long-term effects of stroke.
15 List six general causes of syncope in the geriatric patient.
16 List six general causes of fever in the geriatric patient.
17 Describe the sensations of the three different types of pain.
18 List the signs and symptoms of the following gastrointestinal and abdominal disorders: cholecystitis, hiatal hernia, diverticulitis, appendicitis, peritonitis, kidney stones.
19 Discuss the difference between Type I and Type II diabetes mellitus.
20 List the signs, symptoms, and treatment for insulin shock.
21 List the signs, symptoms, and treatment for diabetic ketoacidosis.
22 Define diabetic retinopathy and diabetic neuropathies.

WORDS TO KNOW

Acclimatization   Becoming accustomed to a change in climate, especially in a warm or hot environment.

Alpha blocker   Chemical or drug that blocks the response of the alpha receptors that vasoconstrict and elevate blood pressure.

Angiotensin converting enzyme   Enzyme in the blood that creates angiotensin, a chemical that causes vasoconstriction and increased blood pressure.

Antidiuretic hormone   Hormone produced by the hypothalamus that decreases the production of urine.

Anticholinergic   Drug that blocks the transmission of nerve impulses in the parasympathetic nervous system.

Aortic stenosis   Cardiac abnormality characterized by the narrowing of the aortic valve. The condition blocks the blood flow out of the left ventricle.

Ascites   Abnormal accumulation of fluid in the abdominal cavity.

Auscultation   Patient assessment technique in which the prehospital care provider listens for sounds inside the body such as breath sounds or heart sounds.

Beta agonists   Chemical or drug that stimulates the beta receptors in the body to increase the heart rate and the force of the heart's contraction. Also increases blood pressure and dilates the arteries and airways.

Beta blocker   Chemical or drug that blocks the stimulation of the beta receptors and slows the heart rate and the heart's force of contraction.

Bruit   Noise caused by turbulence of blood as it passes through a narrowed artery.

Calcium channel blocker   Chemical or drug that blocks the flow of calcium into the muscles. Causes decreased heart rate, along with vasodilation and a decrease in blood pressure.

Cardiomyopathy   Abnormal enlargement of the heart.

Cardioversion   Delivery of a synchronized electric shock to the heart to correct an abnormal heart rhythm such as atrial fibrillation or ventricular tachycardia.

Cholecystitis   Inflammation of the gallbladder. May be accompanied by gallstones.

Chronic obstructive pulmonary disease (COPD)   Condition that includes chronic bronchitis and/or emphysema.

Cilia   Hair-like fibers that line the airways and other special tissues. Produce motion and movement. The cilia help clear the airways of mucus.

Comorbidity   Condition that exists along with another illness.

Defibrillation   Delivery of an electric shock to the heart to correct ventricular fibrillation. Shock is not synchronized to an underlying heart rhythm.

Diaphoresis   Profuse sweating.

Diverticulitis   Inflammation of a pouch-like herniation through the wall of the colon.

Diuretic   Chemical or drug that promotes the excretion of urine.

Dysfunction   Abnormal functioning.

Dysphagia   Difficulty swallowing.

Dysphasia   Difficulty speaking or an impairment of speech.

Dyspnea   Difficulty breathing or shortness of breath.

Dysrhythmia   Abnormal cardiac rhythm or disturbance in the heart's electrical rhythm.

Endocarditis   Inflammation of the inner lining of the heart.

Epidural hematoma   Arterial bleeding in the brain above the dura mater caused by a significant head injury.

Esophageal varicies   Varicose vein in the esophagus.

Fowler's position   Position of the patient when the patient's head is elevated. Usually accompanied by flexion of the knees.

Hemiparesis   Muscle weakness on one side of the body.

Hemiplegia   Paralysis on one side of the body.

Hiatal hernia   Protrusion of the stomach through an opening in the diaphragm.

Homan's sign   Sign of deep vein thrombosis characterized by pain in the calf when the foot is dorsiflexed (upward bending of the foot toward the shin).

Hypertensive encephalopathy   Deterioration of brain functioning including stroke-like symptoms caused by hypertension.

Hypoxic drive   Secondary or backup stimulus to breathe that is generated by low oxygen levels in the blood.

Ketoacidosis   Acidosis (low blood pH) caused by the accumulation of ketones in the body.

Ketones   Products of metabolism of lipids in the liver.

Miliary tuberculosis   Tuberculosis that is widespread or disseminated throughout the body.

Nuchal rigidity   Stiffness of the neck characterized by resistance to flexing of the neck.

Orthostatic hypotension   Significant decrease in blood pressure when the patient is moved from a supine to a sitting or standing position.

Peritonitis   Inflammation of the lining of the abdominal cavity.

Polyarteritis nodosa   Widespread inflammation of small and medium-size arteries. Accompanied by ischemia of the tissue normally served by the inflamed arteries.

Polydipsia   Excessive thirst.

Polyphagia   Excessive hunger or eating.

Polyuria   Excessive urination.

Rales   Abnormal breath sounds caused by air bubbling through fluid. Heard on inspiration.

Rhonchi   Abnormal breath sounds caused by thick secretions or muscle spasms of the airways. Heard on expiration and clear with coughing.

Renal calculi   Accumulation of minerals in the hollow area of the kidney. Also known as kidney stones.

Respiratory acidosis   Acidosis (low body pH) caused by retention of carbon dioxide.

Subarachnoid bleeding   Arterial bleeding deep within the brain that may be caused by a spontaneous rupture of a cerebral artery.

Subdural hematoma   Venous bleeding in the brain below the dura mater, usually after a head injury.

Supraventricular   Originating above the ventricles of the heart.

Syncope   Fainting or brief loss of consciousness usually preceded by a sensation of light-headedness.

Systemic lupus erythematosus   Chronic inflammatory autoimmune disease characterized by injury to the skin, joints, kidneys, and other organs.

Tachydysrhythmia   Abnormally fast heart rate.

Tidal volume   Amount of air inhaled or exhaled with normal breathing.

Vasovagal syncope   Sudden loss of consciousness caused by sudden lack of blood flow to the brain, typically from a sudden drop in blood pressure or cardiac output. Episode is triggered by emotional upset, fear, or trauma.

Vertigo   Sense of rotation or movement of the person or their surroundings.

Prehospital care providers are frequently called on to take care of elderly patients who have a myriad of medical complaints ranging from respiratory ills to accidental injuries. The purpose of this chapter is to focus on the more common complaints found in the elderly. It will begin with a discussion of respiratory emergencies and then present common cardiovascular conditions. Stroke will also be presented, along with information on syncope, fever, gastrointestinal emergencies, diabetes, and heat and cold emergencies. Chapter 9 will discuss commonly encountered injuries in the elderly, including falls, fractures, burns, and decubitus ulcers.

This chapter will only briefly mention some conditions since most EMS textbooks cover them in considerable detail. For example, in the section on cardiovascular emergencies, angina pectoris and acute myocardial infarction are omitted since there is a wealth of information on these conditions in all readily available EMS textbooks.

RESPIRATORY FAILURE AND RESPIRATORY DISTRESS

Respiratory failure is one of the leading causes of death in older adults after cardiovascular disease and cancer. Prehospital care providers will frequently respond to calls where the patient is having trouble breathing. It should be noted that, in spite of advancing age, senior citizens do survive acute episodes of respiratory distress and leave the hospital to return home. This section of the chapter will discuss respiratory distress and acute respiratory failure in the elderly patient. Common respiratory problems seen by prehospital care providers include exacerbations of COPD, respiratory failure, pulmonary embolism, and pneumonia.

As discussed in Chapter 2, the normal changes in aging decrease lung function. Resistance and compliance of the lungs increase, coupled with a drop in vital capacity. If the older adult has an underlying pathological condition such as COPD, the respiratory system can be further impaired.

When assessing a complaint of dyspnea in the elderly, prehospital care providers should remember that dyspnea might be a common complaint associated with aging, and that there may not be any underlying pathology. Thus, a careful and thorough evaluation of the patient is in order.

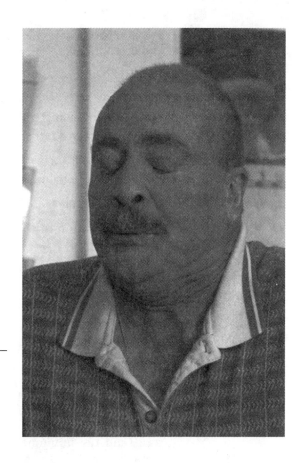

• FIGURE 8-1
Respiratory distress can occur without a history of COPD.

Source: Courtesy Brady *MedEMT,* p. 285.

Chronic Obstructive Pulmonary Disease

Chronic obstructive pulmonary disease (COPD) consists of two diseases, chronic bronchitis and emphysema, with chronic bronchitis as the primary illness. Of the 10 million Americans with COPD, 8 million have chronic bronchitis. Many patients have a combination of both conditions. Asthma may also play a role in COPD.

Patients with chronic bronchitis are called "blue bloaters." The term blue bloater is associated with the clinical presentation of the disease. The predominant feature of chronic bronchitis is excessive mucous production that causes blockage of the airways. Because of damage to the cilia of the airways, clearing the excessive mucus is difficult, causing inflammation of the airways. The pulmonary capillaries are not damaged.

KEY POINT

Blue bloaters are patients with chronic bronchitis. Clinically, they are obese, have noisy breathing caused by excessive mucus in the airways, and are slightly cyanotic. Their primary stimulus to breathe is low oxygen levels in the blood.

The body responds to the chronic bronchitis by increasing the blood flow out of the heart (cardiac output) and decreasing airflow into and out of the alveoli. As a result of poor ventilation, the patient becomes hypoxic and cyanotic.

Arterial carbon dioxide levels increase. Eventually, vasoconstriction of the patient's pulmonary artery leads to a condition known as cor pulmonale, in which the signs and symptoms of right heart failure develop. The resulting edema lends itself to the name, "blue bloater."

Because of chronically increased CO_2 levels in the blood, the principle drive to breathe, carbon dioxide, no longer plays a role in stimulating breathing. Instead, the chronic bronchitic must rely on a secondary mechanism, hypoxic drive, to trigger a breath. When the patient's oxygen levels drop sufficiently, the patient will take a breath.

The signs and symptoms of chronic bronchitis are presented in the following list.

Signs and Symptoms of Chronic Bronchitis

Productive cough

Overweight

Cyanosis

Use of accessory muscles to breathe

Diminished breath sounds with coarse rhonchi

Signs of right heart failure including ascites, jugular vein distention, and pedal edema

In contrast with blue bloaters, emphysema patients have been nicknamed "pink puffers" due to the characteristic signs associated with the disease. Emphysema gradually destroys the walls of the alveoli, the walls dividing these air sacs, and the pulmonary capillaries. The alveoli become stretched and distended as well as scarred. The end result is the inability to diffuse oxygen and carbon dioxide. To compensate, the body reduces its blood flow from the heart, and the patient tends to breathe faster, using puffs to breathe. Because of increased muscle work, the patient will eventually lose weight and experience muscle wasting. Men are more likely to have emphysema than women.

KEY POINT

Emphysema patients are usually thin, use pursed lips to breath, and have a pink color to the skin.

The signs and symptoms of emphysema are presented in the following list.

Signs and Symptoms of Emphysema

Thin body structure

Pursed-lip breathing

Typically found in a sitting or tripod position

Pink or reddened skin

Cyanosis

Use of accessory muscles to breathe

Barrel chest

Wheezing

Decreased breath sounds

Distant heart sounds

Patients with COPD will use bronchodilators and, on occasion, cortico-steroids to treat their condition. These medications can be inhaled in a mist or taken by mouth in a tablet form. The following table lists the various bron-chodilators taken by patients with COPD.

Bronchodilators Taken by Patients with COPD

Type of Drug	Mode of Action	Side Effects	Generic Name (Brand Name)	Method of Administration
Short-acting beta agonists	Stimulate the beta receptors in the lung that relax smooth muscles in the airways. Increase vital capacity and decrease airway resistance.	Tachycardia, tremors, nervousness, irritability, dizziness, headache	Albuterol (Proventil, Ventolin) Metaproterenol (Brethaire) Pirbuterol (Maxair) Isoetharine (Bronkosol)	Metered-dose inhaler, syrup, tablets, nebulized solutions
Long-acting beta agonists	Stimulate the beta receptors in the lung that relax smooth muscles in the airways. Increase vital capacity and decrease airway resistance.	Tachycardia, tremors, nervousness, irritability, dizziness, headache	Albuterol (Proventil Repetabs) Salmeterol (Serevent)	Metered-dose inhaler, orally in table form
Methylxanthine drugs	Act directly on the smooth muscle of the airways and the pulmonary blood vessels. Increase vital capacity and relieve bronchospasm.	Increased heart rate, cardiac dysrhythmia, hypotension, restlessness, irritability	Theophyllin (SloBid, Theo-Dur)	Orally, by capsule, tablet, or syrup
Anticholinergic drugs	Block the action of acetylcholine on bronchial muscles, allowing the airways to dilate.	Dry mouth, blurred vision, tachycardia, headache, decreased urination, confusion	Ipatropium (Atrovent)	Metered-dose inhaler, nebulizer

Patients with COPD can develop exacerbations of the disease and experi-ence acute respiratory failure. The failure is primarily due to the patient's in-ability to maintain adequate diffusion of oxygen and carbon dioxide. The patient will also have problems maintaining an adequate tidal volume of air, thus hypoventilation will contribute to the patient's difficulty breathing. If pulse oximetry is available, the prehospital care provider will see a significant drop in oxygen to a level below 55 mm HG.

> **KEY POINT**
>
> Patients with chronic respiratory diseases may use inhalers to treat acute exacerbations of the disease. Help the patient use their inhaler, and be prepared to administer nebulized medications per local protocol.

Acute Respiratory Failure

As respiratory failure progresses, the patient retains additional carbon dioxide, which leads to a condition known as respiratory acidosis. Respiratory acidosis, in turn, causes additional resistance in the pulmonary blood vessels and dilation of the blood vessels in the brain. Further, the hypoxia can cause deterioration in cardiac function and lead to rhythm disturbances. The patient in respiratory failure will often complain of dyspnea, headache, drowsiness, and confusion. The hypoxic patient may be restless or irritable. Physical examination may reveal shallow breathing, cyanosis, elevated heart rate, and pale, cool, clammy skin. As the condition worsens, the patient may become comatose.

Signs and Symptoms of Acute Respiratory Failure

Headache

Drowsiness

Confusion

Restlessness/irritability

Dyspnea

Shallow breathing

Cyanosis

Tachycardia

Pale, cool, clammy skin

Coma

Treatment of the patient in acute respiratory failure should be aimed at increasing oxygenation of the patient. This can be accomplished by the administration of supplemental oxygen and assisting the patient's breathing. Place the patient in a position of comfort, usually in a semi or full Fowler's position. A sitting position reduces the resistance in the chest and makes ventilation easier. It also reduces the pressure on the diaphragm by the abdominal organs, further reducing resistance in the chest. Administer high-flow, humidified supplemental oxygen. If pulse oximetry is available, try to maintain oxygen levels at 90 percent saturation (SpO_2 90). Monitor the patient's rate and depth of breathing as it may become necessary to intubate and ventilate the patient. Oxygen should be humidified since dry gas can worsen any mucous plugging in the airways. If available, administer a nebulized bronchodilator such as albuterol per local protocol. Monitor the patient's blood pressure and heart rate since the typical bronchodilator used in the field is a beta agonist that can increase heart rate and blood pressure.

To quickly determine if intubation is necessary, have the patient hold the nebulizer in their hand during bronchodilator therapy. If the patient falls asleep or becomes so sleepy that the nebulizer is dropped, then the patient is in need of intubation and assisted ventilation.

If the patient's condition warrants and if it is available, use continuous positive airway pressure (CPAP) or positive end expiratory pressure (PEEP) to assist breathing. Valves that assist in PEEP usually range from 5 to 15 cm of water pressure. Use the lowest setting that achieves the best results, keeping in mind that high PEEP can result in spontaneous pneumothorax, especially in patients with COPD.

Pulmonary Embolism

Not only does COPD pose problems for the older adult, pulmonary embolism can also develop and quickly become life-threatening. Older adults are at higher risk for pulmonary embolism due to several risk factors. These risk factors are presented in the following list.

Risk Factors for Pulmonary Embolism

Burns
Chemotherapy
Congestive heart failure
Fractures
Heart attack
History of deep vein thrombosis or pulmonary embolism
Hormone replacement therapy (estrogen replacement)
Indwelling venous infusion catheters
Lack of mobility (bed ridden)
Malignancy
Obesity
Recent surgery
Recent history of trauma
Systemic lupus erythematosus
Varicose veins with or without venous stasis

Although age alone is not a risk factor, several age-associated conditions place the older adult at a higher risk for pulmonary embolism than younger adults. Studies have shown that pulmonary embolism is often overlooked in the elderly.

Most often, pulmonary embolism is the result of a deep vein thrombosis brought on by any number of factors. The most common sites for the development of a deep vein thrombosis include the calf and pelvic veins, as well as the axillary and subclavian veins. Some studies have shown that deep vein thrombosis that originates in the calf of the leg accounts for 30 to 46 percent of all pulmonary emboli.

KEY POINT

A bed-ridden older adult who has a history of recent injury or surgery is at higher risk for pulmonary embolism.

The signs and symptoms of deep vein thrombosis are mentioned here so that the prehospital care provider will have a better understanding of the overall picture of the patient presenting with pulmonary embolism. It should be noted that not all patients with deep vein thrombosis have any signs or symptoms, and that the assessment of deep vein thrombosis is tenuous at best.

The signs and symptoms of deep vein thrombosis are associated with the amount of obstruction of blood flow and inflammation in the vein. Edema in the area of and below the blockage is a very common finding and is restricted to one leg. Many patients with deep vein thrombosis in the calf will complain of leg pain, especially when the leg is straight and the foot is dorsiflexed (Homan's sign). If the obstruction is in the thigh, the patient may complain of thigh pain. Tenderness may be present in the area of the deep vein thrombosis and the skin may be warm to the touch. A fever may also be present. Patients with a history of deep vein thrombosis may be taking coumadin or other blood thinner. They may also be wearing compression stockings to reduce the chance of clot formation in the legs.

Signs of Deep Vein Thrombosis

Leg or thigh pain

Edema

Tenderness in the area

Homan's sign

Warm skin in the area of blockage (not common)

Unfortunately, pulmonary embolism is often fatal. The condition is responsible for a large number of unexpected deaths annually. It is estimated that 650,000 cases of pulmonary embolism occur in the United States each year. Of those with diagnosed pulmonary embolism, at least 10 percent will die within the first hour of symptom onset.

KEY POINT

Patients with a history of deep vein thrombosis may take anticoagulants and wear compression stockings. Even with these precautions, blood clots in the legs can still develop.

The signs and symptoms of pulmonary embolism include chest pain, tenderness in the chest wall, back and shoulder pain, pain in the upper abdomen, syncope, cough and coughing of blood, dyspnea, and cardiac dysrhythmias. Other findings include hypotension; cor pulmonale (see discussion under COPD); abnormal breath sounds such as wheezing, rales, or diminished breath sounds; tachycardia; profuse sweating; and cyanosis.

Signs and Symptoms of Pulmonary Embolism

Chest pain

Shoulder/back/abdominal pain

Dyspnea

Cough

Hemoptysis

Cardiac dysrhythmias

Tachycardia

Hypotension

Shock

Diaphoresis

Cyanosis

Pedal edema

Abnormal breath sounds (wheezes, rales, absent sounds)

Cardiac arrest

Prehospital care of patients with a pulmonary embolism should be aimed at prompt stabilization of the patient and transportation to the nearest emergency department. Since making an absolute diagnosis of pulmonary embolism in the field is extremely difficult, a specific treatment plan is equally difficult to develop.

High-flow oxygen and ventilatory support, including intubation, should be initiated along with an IV access line. Patients in shock may not benefit from fluid loading, thus fluid resuscitation should be reserved for those whose condition is quickly deteriorating. If available, monitor the patient's ECG and pulse oximetry.

KEY POINT

Treatment of pulmonary embolism includes high flow oxygen, ventilatory assistance, and an IV. Monitor the patient's ECG and pulse oximetry.

If it is known that the patient has a history of or is being treated for a deep vein thrombosis, the emergency department physician may order the administration of a clot-busting medication such as tPA (tissue plasminogen activator).

Follow local basic life support and advanced cardiac life support protocols for patients in cardiac arrest. Keep in mind that prompt transportation to the emergency department will increase the chances of survival for patients with pulmonary embolism.

Bacterial Pneumonia

Bacterial pneumonia is another serious illness the elderly patient may contract. Over 60,000 deaths occur each year from pneumonia. Generally speaking, aging increases the risk of mortality from pneumonia. Pneumonia is the fourth or fifth leading cause of death in the elderly. For this reason, older adults are encouraged to receive a pneumococcus vaccination in conjunction with the annual flu shot.

The principal cause of bacterial pneumonia bacteria from the upper airway that migrate into the lungs. If the immune system fails to destroy the bacteria, they will invade the body and the patient will succumb to the infection. Risk factors for developing pneumonia include poor immune system response because of aging and impairment of the normal body defense mechanisms caused by conditions such as COPD, cancer, inhaled toxins, or aspiration.

Once the infection develops and is left untreated, it can damage the lungs by scarring the lung tissue. This reduces the number of alveoli able to participate in oxygen-carbon dioxide exchange. An initial infection can lead to subsequent and sequential infections that further impair the body's respiratory and immune systems.

Patients with pneumonia may have signs and symptoms that range from mild or minimal to severe and life-threatening. One sign of pneumonia is a productive cough. The sputum color or odor depends on the infectious organism and may range from rust colored (Pneumococcus) to green (Pseudomonas, Hemophilus, and Pneumococcus) to the color of currant jelly (Klebsiella and Pneumococcus). Foul-smelling sputum may be indicative of infection by anaerobic bacteria.

The patient is often febrile with shaking chills. The patient may complain of chest discomfort or pain, headache, uneasiness, nausea, vomiting, muscle aches and pain, exertional dyspnea, anorexia, or weight loss. Additionally, the patient may be breathing rapidly accompanied by an increased or slowed heart rate. Cyanosis along with hypotension and altered mental status may be present if hypoxia is severe. Auscultation of the chest may reveal decreased breath sounds in the affected areas along with wheezing, rhonchi, and rales. Tapping on or percussing the chest will produce a dull sound. The following list presents the signs and symptoms of pneumonia.

Signs and Symptoms of Pneumonia

Chest pain/discomfort
Productive cough
Headache
Uneasiness
Nausea/vomiting
Muscle aches and pain
Dyspnea and dyspnea on exertion
Increased breathing
Tachycardia or bradycardia
Hypotension
Abnormal breath sounds (wheezing, rales, rhonchi)
Altered mental status

In the prehospital setting, treatment of patients with pneumonia is based upon the degree of respiratory distress. After placing the patient in a position of comfort, mild distress is best treated with the administration of supplemental oxygen based on the patient's needs. For those patients in respiratory failure, positive pressure ventilation along with intubation, if available, may be necessary to ensure adequate oxygenation. Since many older adults with pneumonia are also dehydrated, the prehospital care provider should initiate IV therapy with lactated Ringer's or a normal saline solution.

> ### KEY POINT
>
> Older adults are highly susceptible to pneumonia during the cold and flu season. Administer oxygen and support breathing as needed.

CARDIOVASCULAR EMERGENCIES

Cardiovascular emergencies, particularly angina pectoris and myocardial infarction, are fairly well covered in prehospital care provider textbooks, and therefore they will not be covered here. However, many elderly patients have underlying cardiovascular diseases and other medical conditions can complicate the care of the acute emergency cardiac episode. There are three conditions that will be discussed in this section. These conditions, which are frequently found in the elderly patient, include hypertension, along with hypertensive crisis; heart failure; and aortic dissection. Deep vein thrombosis, although a cardiovascular disease, was discussed in the section on respiratory emergencies since it is related to pulmonary embolism. In addition to these emergency conditions, this section will present information pertaining to implanted pacemakers and automatic internal cardiac defibrillators.

Hypertension and Hypertensive Crisis

Hypertension is defined as a persistent elevation of systolic and/or diastolic blood pressure. The elevation is such that organ damage can occur if it is not treated. An old rule of thumb states that normal systolic blood pressure for the adult can be estimated using the following guideline:

$$\frac{100 + \text{age of individual}}{70\text{--}80}$$

The maximum should be 140/90.

The blood pressure tends to increase with age. Around the age of 60 years, the diastolic pressure tends to stabilize even though the systolic pressure may continue to increase. In the United States, statistics show that over 50 percent of those over the age of 65 years have been diagnosed with hypertension. Until recently, an elevated diastolic pressure was considered a key risk factor toward the development of hypertension-related diseases. The role of the diastolic pressure, although important, has been downplayed in recent years. Patients with an elevated systolic blood pressure of 160 mm Hg or higher were thought to be at significant risk of complications. Currently, that number has been revised downward to a systolic blood pressure of 140 mm Hg or higher. Evidence has suggested that the risk of heart attack or stroke is significantly higher when the systolic pressure, not the diastolic, is elevated.

In 1993, the Joint Committee on Detection, Evaluation, and Treatment of High Blood Pressure established a classification of hypertension. The following table shows the classification of hypertension.

Classification		Systolic Pressure (mm Hg)	Diastolic Pressure (mm Hg)
Normal		<130	<85
High normal		130–139	85–89
Hypertension	Stage 1 (mild)	140–159	90–99
	Stage 2 (moderate)	160–179	100–109
	Stage 3 (severe)	180–209	109–119
	Stage 4 (very severe)	≥210	≥120

KEY POINT

A blood pressure over 140/90 is hypertensive.

The end result of hypertension can be severe. Patients with untreated hypertension have developed heart failure, stroke, peripheral vascular disease, and kidney failure. After a diagnosis of hypertension, patients will often take a regimen of medications designed to lower the systolic and diastolic pressures. The prehospital care provider should be aware of the classifications and names of antihypertensive medications the geriatric patient may be taking. The following table lists the drug classifications and the names of frequently prescribed antihypertensive drugs.

KEY POINT

When assessing a patient, ask about any medications they may be taking. Also ask the patient if they know why they are taking a specific drug. Be alert for medications that are used to treat hypertension.

Hypertensive crisis is an acute emergency that prehospital care providers may encounter in the field. Instead of an actual blood pressure measurement, hypertensive emergencies are based on the damage to target organs. For example, consider conditions such as hypertensive encephalopathy, heart attack, congestive heart failure, unstable angina, and dissection of the aorta. Since hypertension may be associated with an underlying condition, the prehospital care provider should assess for an associated pathology and treat the patient accordingly. For example, a patient with an acute hypertensive emergency may be hypoglycemic. Treating the low blood sugar could alleviate the hypertension.

KEY POINT

Hypertensive crisis is not so much the actual blood pressure, but the damage the high blood pressure is doing to the organs.

Drug Classification	Generic Name (Brand Name)
Diuretics	Chlorothiazide (Diuril)
	Hydrochlorothiazide (Hydrodiuril)
	Furosemide (Lasix)
	Spironolactone (Aldactone)
Alpha Blockers	Clonidine (Catapres)
	Doxazosin (Cardura)
	Methyldopa (Aldomet)
	Prazosin (Minipres)
	Reserpine (Serpalan)
	Terazosin (Hytrin)
Beta Blockers	Atenolol (Tenormin)
	Labetalol (Trandate)
	Metoprolol (Lopressor)
	Nadolol (Corgard)
	Propranolol (Inderal)
Vasodilators	Hydrazaline (Apresoline)
Calcium channel blockers	Amlodipine (Norvasc)
	Diltiazem (Cardizem)
	Felodipine (Plendil)
	Nicardipine (Cardene)
	Nifedipine (Adalat, Procardia)
	Verapamil (Calan)
Angiotensin converting enzyme (ACE) inhibitors	Benazepril (Lotensin)
	Captopril (Capoten)
	Enalapril (Vasotec)
	Lisinopril (Prinivil)
	Quinapril (Accupril)
	Ramipril (Altace)

Patients with acute hypertensive emergencies could suffer hypertensive encephalopathy. This condition puts the patient at risk of death from prolonged and severe elevations of blood pressure. Signs and symptoms of hypertensive encephalopathy include headache, nausea, vomiting, stroke-like symptoms, blindness, seizures, coma, and, ultimately, death. Recognizing the condition is critical since the patient needs medication to lower the blood pressure as well as prompt transportation to the emergency department.

Prehospital treatment of hypertensive crisis consists of elevating the patient's head or placing the patient in a position of comfort, administering high-flow oxygen, starting an IV of D5W, and monitoring the patient's ECG. In severe cases, the emergency department physician may order the sublingual administration of nifedipine or nitroglycerin to dilate the patient's blood vessels and lower the blood pressure. Other medications used to treat hypertensive emergencies include sodium nitroprusside (Nipride), labetalol (Trandate), and morphine sulfate. Care must be taken not to lower the patient's blood pressure too much. Monitor the patient carefully and, if the patient develops conditions associated with or aggravated by the high blood pressure such as pulmonary edema from congestive heart failure, treat the patient accordingly.

Congestive Heart Failure

Heart failure, both acute and chronic, occurs frequently in the elderly population. Congestive heart failure is defined as the failure of one or more of the heart's chambers to function properly. The result is a backing up of fluid into either the lungs or the systemic circulation. The more common causes of the disorder include hypertension and coronary artery disease. Usually the left ventricle fails first, frequently followed by the failure of the right ventricle. Left heart failure can be precipitated in the older population by cardiac valve problems such as stenosis of the aortic valve and mitral regurgitation. Certain dysrhythmias such as atrial fibrillation can contribute to left heart failure as well.

In the early stages of left heart failure, the patient may complain of dyspnea that occurs only at night (nocturnal dyspnea) or shortness of breath that is relieved by sitting (orthopnea). The patient may also complain of a dry cough that worsens at night. As the condition deteriorates, the patient will eventually develop pulmonary edema that can be heard as rales or rhonchi when auscultating lung sounds. It should be noted that in the older adult, rales can be caused by a number of conditions, including heart failure, pulmonary fibrosis, or COPD. The fine crackles or rales need to be interpreted cautiously. However, a patient in full left heart failure will typically present in a fully upright position and complain of severe dyspnea. The following list presents the signs and symptoms of left heart failure.

Signs and Symptoms of Left Heart Failure

Sitting upright
Severe dyspnea
Use of accessory muscles to breathe
Coughing a pink, frothy sputum
Bilateral rales, occasionally heard in all lung fields
Cyanosis
Profuse diaphoresis
Chest pain may or may not be present

KEY POINT

Be suspicious of a patient who complains of difficulty breathing at night or dyspnea that is relieved by sitting. Both are early warnings of congestive heart failure.

Treatment for left heart failure includes proper positioning of the patient and administering high-flow oxygen. Place the patient in a Fowler's position and, if possible, allow the patient's feet to dangle off the stretcher. The sitting position reduces pressure on the patient's back and reduces the resistance inside the chest. Decreasing the pressure of the abdominal organs on the diaphragm also reduces resistance inside the chest. Finally, elevating the patient's head moves the fluids in the alveoli to the lung bases, allowing better ventilation of the alveoli in the upper lung fields. Having the legs dangle from the side of the stretcher will reduce venous return to the heart.

Administer high-flow oxygen while monitoring the rate and depth of ventilation, especially in patients with underlying COPD. If necessary, assist breathing with intermittent positive pressure and, if required and available, intubate the patient. Advanced life-support care includes monitoring the ECG, initiating IV therapy, and administering medications to relieve the fluid in the alveoli. Drugs that are typically used in the prehospital treatment of left heart failure include nitroglycerin, furosemide, and morphine sulfate. Cardiac drugs may be needed if the patient develops cardiogenic shock.

Dissecting Aortic Aneurysm

Acute aortic dissection is a critical condition that can lead to the patient's death in a matter of minutes should the dissection lead to rupture. A dissecting aortic aneurysm is caused by a tear in the lining of the aorta that allows bleeding into the walls of the blood vessel. An aortic aneurysm is primarily caused by hypertension. In the elderly, the most common site for an aortic aneurysm is in the descending aorta after the blood vessel curves downward from the arch (see the following illustration).

Signs and symptoms of aortic dissection can vary, but typically include back pain that may radiate throughout the chest and back. In some cases, pain is absent. Depending upon the location of the aneurysm, peripheral pulses may be varied. Additionally, if blood flow to vital organs such as the kidneys or intestines is blocked, abdominal or flank pain may be a presenting symptom. This sign is strongly suggestive of an aortic aneurysm because of the multiple areas of pain caused by a loss of blood flow to vital tissues. Depending on the size and location of the aneurysm along with the resulting blood clot formed by the bleeding, a pulsating (pulsatile) mass may be felt in the abdomen.

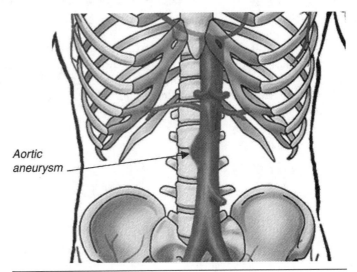

Aortic aneurysm

• FIGURE 8-2
Aortic aneurysm occurs when the aorta bulges like a balloon.
A rupture could be fatal.
Source: Courtesy Brady *MedEMT,* p. 124.

Prehospital care of the dissecting aneurysm is oriented toward prompt transportation to the emergency department. High-flow supplemental oxygen should be provided and, where available, two large-bore IVs of either normal saline or lactated Ringer's solution should be started. Prehospital care providers should apply the pneumatic antishock garment if available and, per protocol, inflate as needed. Since this condition is a surgical emergency, rapid transportation to a receiving hospital with a surgical team is warranted.

Pacemakers and Automatic Internal Cardiac Defibrillators

With aging or with myocardial infarction, the heart's electrical circuit can deteriorate, causing the heart's rate to slow significantly. At times, the heart rate may decrease to a point where the patient is at risk of passing out from the lack of blood flow to the brain. Other organs may also be at risk of damage due to reduced blood flow.

To compensate for the slow heart rhythm, physicians implant a pacemaker into the patient's chest with lead wires attached to the inner lining of patient's heart. The pacemaker is set in one of two modes—synchronous (fixed rate) or asynchronous (demand). In the fixed-rate mode, the pacemaker is set to fire at a set rate without regard to the heart's electrical activity or rate. In the demand mode, the pacemaker is programmed to generate a pulse if it does not sense any electrical activity for a specified period of time. When a pacemaker pulse is generated, a spike will be noted on the patient's ECG (see illustration).

Conditions in which a pacemaker may be implanted include:

Sick sinus syndrome accompanied by symptomatic sinus bradycardia

Atrial fibrillation with a slow ventricular response

Complete heart block

Inadequate heart rate to compensate for demand (exercise)

Cardiomyopathy

Paroxysmal atrial fibrillation

A device similar to the pacemaker called the Automatic Internal Cardiac Defibrillator (ICD) has been designed to sense a rapid ventricular heartbeat and, when necessary, administer a shock to cardiovert or defibrillate the patient. It may also be programmed to fire rapidly for a number of paces in an attempt to end an episode of ventricular tachycardia. Both the pacemaker and the ICD are designed to correct potentially life-threatening heart rhythms. Newer devices on the market contain a combination pacemaker and ICD, and are used in patients who need the capabilities of both devices.

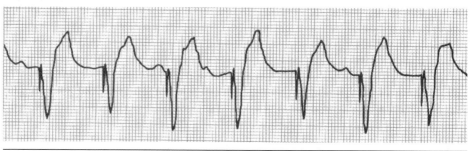

• FIGURE 8-3

Pacemaker generated rhythm.

Source: Courtesy Brady *Paramedic Emergency Care,* 3rd ed., p. 672.

Prehospital care providers should be alert to potential problems with pacemakers and ICD devices. There are several pacemaker complications that prehospital care providers may encounter in the field. These include output failure, failure to capture, oversensing, and undersensing.

Output failure occurs when the pacemaker fails to generate a pulse even though there is reason to pace. Evidence of this failure would be seen on the ECG as the absence of a pacemaker spike in a bradycardia. Causes for the failure to output include battery failure, a broken lead, oversensing, or poor lead connection. In the event of output failure, the prehospital care provider may have to provide advanced cardiac life support (ACLS) based on the proper protocol for the bradycardia. Follow ACLS or local protocols in treating the symptomatic bradycardia.

Failure to capture is another complication that can be caused by a broken lead, myocardial infarction at the lead tip, medications, or poor lead connection. Evidence of failure to capture is seen on the ECG as a pacemaker spike that is not followed by a QRS (ventricular) complex. Treatment for failure to capture is similar to that for output failure and is based on the patient's needs.

KEY POINT

A patient with a broken pacemaker lead may develop a profound bradycardia and require immediate intervention.

Oversensing occurs when the pacemaker senses electrical activity that blocks the generation of a pacemaker pulse. Muscular activity of the heart, diaphragm, or pectoral muscles can cause oversensing. This complication may or may not be encountered in the prehospital setting. However, should a patient present with oversensing as a part of their chief complaint, the prehospital care provider needs to assess and treat the patient's heart rate and associated symptoms.

Undersensing is when the pacemaker fails to recognize electrical activity and generates a pulse in spite of the heart's own cardiac rhythm. Treatment for this condition is the same as that for output failure and failure to capture.

Complications of ICD devices include failures similar to those found in pacemakers, inappropriate cardioversion or defibrillation, and deactivation of the device. In a combination device, the ICD may also exhibit output failure and failure to capture.

Undersensing with an ICD may occur when the programmed rate to cardiovert ventricular tachycardia is set too high. If the programmed sense is set at 180 and the episode or ventricular tachycardia is 160, there will be no cardioversion. Paramedics may need to follow ACLS or local protocols in treating the patient's ventricular tachycardia.

Oversensing occurs when the ICD delivers a shock in the absence of a lethal cardiac rhythm. At times, ICDs have recognized atrial fibrillation with a rapid ventricular rate as a lethal rhythm and delivered a shock. Causes of oversensing other than atrial fibrillation may include broken leads or electromagnetic interference such as that caused by an MRI.

STROKE

Stroke, also known as cerebrovascular accident or brain attack, is a devastating illness that affects between 500,000 to 600,000 people in the United States each year. Of that number, up to 150,000 people die from stroke, making it the third leading cause of death in the country. Stroke is also the leading cause of disability in the United States.

Regardless of the name, the effects are the same—significant damage to the brain with lasting disability that can drastically impair the victim's quality of life. A stroke is caused by the sudden interruption of blood flow to a part of the brain. There are three causes of a stroke: a blood clot or embolism, a ruptured blood vessel, and blood supply problems outside of the brain (shock). The following table highlights the incidence of the primary causes of stroke.

Primary Causes of Stroke

Cause	Frequency (percent)
Bleeding	25
Thrombosis/embolism	75

KEY POINT

A majority of strokes in the older population are caused by blood clots.

In order to understand how a stroke affects the patient, it is important to review the anatomy and physiology of the brain. The brain has been described as a mass of soft, spongy tissue that appears pinkish gray in color. It weighs an average of 3 pounds and consists of three main structures—the cerebrum, the cerebellum, and the brain stem. The largest of these structures is the cerebrum, which is responsible for high levels of thought, emotions, intellectual functioning, speech, interpretation of sensory input, and control of fine movement. The cerebrum consists of the cerebral cortex, which is also known as the "gray matter." Beneath the gray matter is a network of nerve fibers that allow the different parts of the brain to communicate with itself.

The cerebral cortex is divided into two halves, or hemispheres, by a long, deep valley (fissure) that runs from the front to the back of the brain. Deep inside the fissure is the corpus callosum, matted white fibers that connect the two hemispheres of the brain allowing each side to communicate and process information. Each hemisphere controls the functions on the opposite side of the body. Thus, the left hemisphere of the cerebral cortex controls the right side of the body and the right hemisphere controls the left side of the body.

Areas of the cerebral cortex have been identified as controlling certain functions of the body. The following illustration highlights some of the functions of specific regions of the cerebral cortex.

Beneath the cerebral cortex are two important centers—the thalamus and the hypothalamus. The thalamus serves as a relay station for sensations received by the body. The thalamus is the principal site where pain is felt.

Below the thalamus is the hypothalamus, which participates in many of the body's vital functions. The hypothalamus regulates the body's fluids, metabolism, blood sugar levels, and temperature. It also controls the body's rhythmic cycles, including rest and activity, sexual desire, and the menstrual and reproductive cycles. Finally, the hypothalamus is known as the integrating center of the autonomic nervous system responsible for the fight or flight response and the slowing of bodily functions.

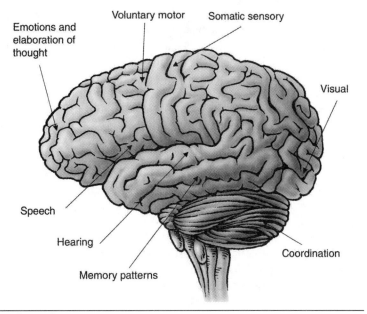

Emotions and elaboration of thought

Voluntary motor

Somatic sensory

Visual

Speech

Hearing

Memory patterns

Coordination

• FIGURE 8-4

Damage to key functional centers of the brain will produce deficits in those functions.

Source: Courtesy Brady *MedEMT,* p. 133.

The second structure of the brain, the cerebellum, is also referred to as the "little brain." The cerebellum is located at the back of the brain, under the curve of the cerebrum. Its function is to coordinate voluntary muscle movement and maintain balance. Although it does not direct movement, the cerebellum allows movements to be smooth and coordinated.

KEY POINT

A cerebellar stroke can result in a lack of coordination that may increase the risk of falling.

The third structure of the brain, the brain stem, consists of the midbrain, medulla oblongata, and the pons. The brain stem serves to connect the cerebral hemispheres with the spinal cord. The brain stem is responsible for the vegetative functions such as breathing, blood vessel control, and heart rate. Additionally, the brainstem is responsible for wakefulness, arousal, and attention. In the medulla oblongata, the sensory input from the body and the motor control over the body's movements cross over from left to right and right to left. The mechanism and reasons for this switchover are not understood.

The brain demands oxygen and carbohydrates to maintain its high level of functioning. The circulation to the brain is provided by two major sets of blood vessels—the common carotid arteries and the vertebral arteries. The common carotid arteries have two main divisions. The first division, the external carotid arteries, provide blood flow to the face and scalp. The second division, the internal carotid arteries, supplies blood flow to the forward-most sections of the cerebrum. The vertebral arteries supply the back sections of the brain along with the brain stem and parts of the cerebellum.

The internal carotid arteries and the vertebral arteries form a circle of arteries at the base of the brain. This structure is known as the Circle of Willis from which other arteries arise and travel to the parts of the brain (see illustration). The other arteries that supply blood to the brain from the Circle of Willis are the anterior cerebral artery, middle cerebral artery, and posterior cerebral artery. One of the nice features of the Circle of Willis is if one of the main arteries is occluded, the smaller arteries that are supplied by that blocked blood vessel can still receive blood from the other main arteries. This function is known as collateral circulation.

From the Circle of Willis, the anterior cerebral artery moves up and forward to bring blood to the frontal lobes of the brain. The posterior cerebral artery supplies the temporal and occipital lobes of the brain. The middle cerebral artery extends into the middle of the brain and branches into deep penetrating arteries that supply blood to the central structures. It is estimated that 20 percent of the strokes occur in these smaller branches.

There are several risk factors associated with strokes. These are the same risk factors that are associated with heart disease and heart attack. The following list summarizes the risk factors for a stroke.

Risk Factors for Stroke

Hypertension
Diabetes
Heart disease
Smoking
Obesity
Elevated cholesterol/lipids
Sedentary lifestyle
Excessive use of alcohol
Use of illicit drugs

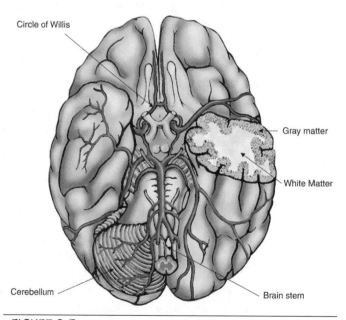

• FIGURE 8-5
Structures of the brain including the circle of Willis.
Source: Courtesy Brady *MedEMT,* p. 429.

Aging (over 60 years of age)
Male
Heredity

When a stroke occurs, there is a decrease in or blockage in blood flow to a portion of the brain. The flow of blood is inadequate to permit normal brain functions from continuing. The result is death or significant damage to the affected brain tissues. As mentioned earlier, there are three principal causes of a stroke: a blood clot, a ruptured blood vessel, and drop in the blood supply to the brain from a cause outside of the brain. Differentiating the cause of a stroke is at times difficult. A stroke that comes on while at rest, during sleep, or when arising from sleep, suggests a blood clot. A stroke that develops after exertion that may be accompanied by headache, stupor, coma, severe hypertension, and seizures suggests a hemorrhage. Regardless of the cause, the end result is cerebrovascular insufficiency.

KEY POINT

A stroke that occurs during rest or sleep suggests a blood clot, whereas a stroke that follows exertion suggests a hemorrhage.

If a blood clot forms, it could develop in one of the brain's arteries and block normal blood flow. Narrowing of the cerebral artery from atherosclerosis may cause this clot (thrombus). A second type of blood clot is one that is formed outside the brain. The clot may break free and travel to the cerebral artery where it becomes lodged. This "floating" clot, or embolus, frequently forms in the heart because of a rhythm disturbance (atrial fibrillation). The clot then travels to the brain where it lodges and causes a stroke. Prehospital care providers who find a patient with obvious signs and symptoms of a stroke and find that the patient has an irregular heart rhythm should suspect atrial fibrillation as the cause of the clot and the stroke.

Strokes may also be caused when an artery in the brain ruptures. Occasionally, a small cerebral artery develops an aneurysm that bursts with elevated blood pressure or other precipitating factors.

Another cause of a stroke is an interruption in blood flow to the brain from a cause outside of the brain. For example, shock can cause a reduction in blood flow to the brain resulting in cerebrovascular insufficiency. If allowed to continue for a prolonged period, brain damage occurs.

KEY POINT

Any prolonged interruption in blood flow to the brain, even from causes outside of the brain, can result in stroke or serious brain damage.

The result of a stroke is damage to a portion of the brain. The signs and symptoms of a stroke vary depending on where the stroke occurs and the extent of the damage. The signs and symptoms of a stroke include the following.

Dizziness

Confusion

Severe headache

Hemiparesis (weakness on one side of the body)

Hemiplegia (paralysis on one side of the body)

Facial droop

Dysphagia (difficulty swallowing)

Drooling

Numbness or altered sensation on one side of the body

Blurred vision or loss of vision

Difficulty in walking

Lack of coordination in the arms and hands

Dysphasia (difficulty speaking)

Dyspnea

Deviated gaze

Seizures—focal or general

Pale, cool clammy skin

Hypertension during the initial stages

There are a few diagnostic tools available for use in prehospital care. One such tool, the Mini Mental Status Exam was discussed in the chapter on Alzheimer's disease. This tool can be used to identify cognitive weaknesses caused by the stroke.

Another tool is the Cincinnati Prehospital Stroke Scale. It is a three-point scale that helps identify a stroke in the prehospital setting. It is especially useful when the signs and symptoms of the stroke are mild and could be overlooked. The following illustration shows the Cincinnati Prehospital Stroke Scale.

KEY POINT

A quick assessment for stroke includes looking for facial droop, arm drift, and abnormal speech (Cincinnati Stroke Scale).

Another tool that may be adaptable to prehospital care is the National Institute of Health Stroke Scale (NIHSS). It is a more detailed description of the stroke's signs and symptoms and, due to time constraints, it may not be an ideal evaluation tool for prehospital care providers. A copy of the NIHSS is included in the appendix for reference.

If the signs and symptoms of a stroke resolve within 24 hours, the patient has actually experienced a transient ischemic attack (TIA). A TIA, often referred to as a mini-stroke is a condition in which the blood flow to the brain is interrupted for a short period of time, then restored. Usually, the TIA lasts for 5 to 20 minutes, however, the symptoms can last for just under 24 hours. The signs and symptoms of a TIA are the same as for a stroke.

KEY POINT

A TIA is a temporary stroke in which the signs and symptoms resolve completely in less than 24 hours. It is a warning that a stroke is pending.

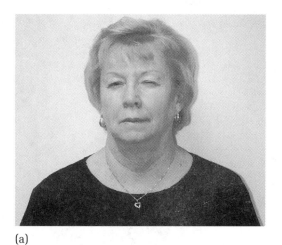

(a)

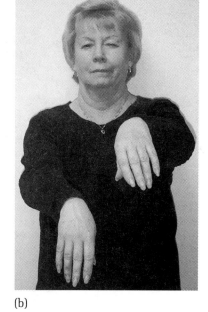

(b)

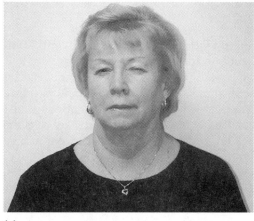

(c)

• FIGURE 8-6

Stroke scale: (a) Facial droop. Normal: both sides of the face move equally. Abnormal: one side of face does not move. (b) Arm drift. Normal: both arms move equally. Abnormal: one arm drifts and is not held equal. (c) Speech. Normal: uses correct words, no slurring. Abnormal: slurred speech, inappropriate words.

In a real stroke, the duration of the signs and symptoms depends on how quickly blood flow to the brain can be restored. If blood flow can quickly be returned to normal, the signs and symptoms may resolve within minutes to hours. However, the longer the period without blood flow, the more severe and permanent the symptoms become. If the brain is permanently damaged, the patient may suffer from a permanent disability.

Prehospital care for the patient with a stroke includes the ABCs of basic life support. In many cases, the patient can be placed in a position of comfort, usually with their head elevated, and transported to the hospital. In cases of extreme hypertension, elevating the patient's head may help to slightly reduce the pressure. The use of oxygen in the uncomplicated case is controversial since oxygen can increase blood pressure by constricting the arteries. Follow local protocol pertaining to the use of oxygen in acute care of the stroke patient.

Patients who are having minimal trouble breathing (dyspnea) should be placed in a semi-Fowler's position and administered oxygen. Those who are dyspneic and are having trouble with their secretions should be placed on the affected side with their head slightly lower than the body. Placing the patient on the affected side removes any weight from the "good" side, facilitates

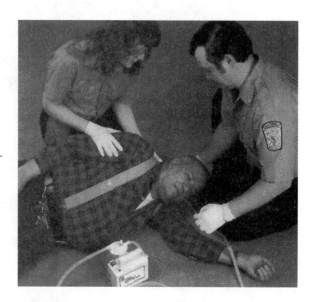

• FIGURE 8-7
Place an unconscious stroke patient in the left lateral recumbent (recovery) position to help keep the airway clear. Suction any secretions as necessary.
Source: Courtesy Brady *Emergency Care,* 8th ed., p. 804.

drainage, and allows easier expansion and ventilation of the unaffected lung. Remember to suction the airway as necessary.

Advanced life-support measures may include antihypertensive therapy, anticonvulsant medications, and endotracheal intubation. Some EMS systems have begun administering clot-dissolving medications such as tPA, however prehospital use of this drug is not recommended. Clot-dissolving medications must be given within a 3-hour window (3 hours from symptom onset), and should not be administered to the patient with a stroke caused by a ruptured artery. It is important to get the patient to a medical center where they can be accurately diagnosed and begin stroke therapy as early as possible. With early intervention and prompt rehabilitation, the long-term effects of the stroke can be minimized.

With a large number of older adults suffering from strokes each year, EMS will be called on to assist some of those patients with the debilitating long-term effects of a stroke. Some of these disabilities will affect the patient's quality of life and could put them at risk for injuries. The following table lists the long-term disabilities that can result from a stroke.

KEY POINT

Long-term disabilities from a stroke are numerous and pose a challenge to the patient as well as their caregivers. Early recognition and intervention in stroke care are essential in reducing the residual effects and disabilities of the disease.

Patients with stroke are a challenge to themselves, their caregivers, and to the prehospital care providers called to provide care during the acute phase and, later, for related problems during and after recovery.

SYNCOPE

Frequently, prehospital care providers will receive calls from elderly patients who complain of weakness or dizziness. Although the patient does not know what caused the episode, they may give a history of suddenly passing out or feeling like they will pass out.

Disability	Affect on Quality of Life
Hemiparesis or hemiplegia	Increased risk of falls. May be bed-bound or wheelchair-bound with increased risk of decubitus ulcers as well as pneumonia.
Loss of balance/coordination	Increased risk of falls.
Dysphasia or dysarthria	Trouble understanding language or speaking. Cannot communicate effectively.
Bodily neglect or inattention	Increased risk of injury. Inadequate nutrition because of inability to feed self or see some food.
Pain, numbness, altered sensation	May have contracted arms or legs. May not be able to sense when injured. Can develop infections more easily.
Problems with memory, thinking	Cannot provide self-care. May require a caregiver.
Problem with attention, learning	Forgets simple things, may be at risk for injury such as that from a stove or oven left on and unattended.
Denial	Patient denies or ignores the effects of the stroke and may attempt to drive while physically impaired.
Dysphagia	Increased risk for malnutrition and dehydration. May also tend to choke.
Incontinence	May need assistance with toilet habits and may soil him or herself frequently. If left unsanitary, skin breakdown can occur. In some cases, patients may be catheterized and, as such, may be at a high risk for urinary tract infections.
Easily fatigued	Risk for losing independence and not being able to perform self-care.
Emotional outbursts	Suddenly cries, yells, laughs, or is angry for no particular reason. This is also seen in multi-infarct dementia.
Depression	Very common in patients with stroke. May lead to suicide ideation or suicide.

Syncope, or a sudden, temporary loss of consciousness, has a number of causes and, when seen in the elderly patient, requires an investigation as to its cause. While many older adults do not actually lose consciousness, they may feel extremely weak or dizzy. This presyncope causes lightheadedness that can be frightening to the senior, and they may call 9-1-1 for help. Although most episodes of syncope are not dangerous, some may be ominous and herald a life-threatening event.

When a patient presents with syncope, prehospital care providers need to perform a thorough history and patient assessment to determine the nature of the loss of consciousness, and then provide treatment and transportation of the patient as needed.

KEY POINT

Syncope or dizziness without loss of consciousness indicates a potentially serious problem in the older adult and requires a thorough patient assessment.

The causes of syncope or presyncope are numerous and can be divided into cardiac and noncardiac reasons. The following lists highlight the various causes of syncope.

Cardiovascular Causes of Syncope

Dysrhythmias
> Bradycardia
> Sinus arrest
> Heart block including second- and third-degree heart block
> Atrial fibrillation with a slow ventricular rate
> Atrial fibrillation with inadequate cardiac output
> Supraventricular tachycardia
> Ventricular tachycardia

Structure Abnormalities
> Aortic stenosis
> Cardiac enlargement
> Pulmonary hypertension
> Myocardial infarction

Noncardiac Causes of Syncope

Vasomotor tone
> Vasovagal syncope
> Orthostatic hypotension
> Carotid sinus hypersensitivity
> Coughing
> Swallowing
> Urination
> Defecation

Drug-related causes
> Hypotension
> Tachycardia
> Bradycardia
> Overdose

Heat-related casues
> Heat exhaustion
> Heat stroke

Cerebrovascular causes
> Stroke
> Hemorrhage
> Seizure

A guide for evaluating the causes of syncope was developed by Dr. Bill Young at the University of Kentucky at Lexington. He suggests using the acronyms HEAD, HEART, and VESSELS to guide in assessing a syncopal episode. (Lists are presented courtesy of Mind-Sharpeners, www.erworld.com).

HEAD—Causes Related to the Central Nervous System

H   Hypoglycemia or hypoxia
E   Epilepsy
A   Anxiety
D   Dysfunction of the brain stem

HEART—Causes Related to the Heart

H   Heart attack

E   Embolism such as pulmonary embolism

A   Aortic stenosis (in the elderly)

R   Rhythm disturbance

T   Tachycardias, including ventricular and supraventricular tachycardia

VESSELS—Causes Related to the Blood Vessels

V   Vasovagal syncope (common fainting)

E   Ectopic pregnancy (unlikely in the elderly, but reminds of hypovolemia)

S   Situational factors, including urination, defecation, and cough syncope

S   Subclavian steal

E   Ears, nose, and throat, including syncope associated with swallowing

L   Low SVR as seen in diabetic neuropathy

S   Sensitive carotid sinus

When confronted with a patient who complains of "passing out," the prehospital care provider needs to carefully assess the patient and perform a detailed history and physical examination. Prior to making contact with the patient, the prehospital care provider will observe the overall scene, looking for hazards to the patient and the EMS crew while also searching for clues pertaining to the current medical problem. The prehospital care provider may tend to overlook some subtle environmental factors that may have led to the patient's syncope. When entering a private home, consider the ambient temperature. A cold or overly warm house could hint at hypo- or hyperthermia as the underlying cause of the syncope.

The prehospital care provider should ask about the patient's past medical history as well as the history of the present illness. Question the patient about any medications they may be taking, taking particular note of any new medications they have recently started. Questions should also include over-the-counter preparations (NSAIDs or herbal remedies). Of particular importance is asking the patient about diabetes. Patients with Type I or Type II diabetes can experience hypoglycemic episodes and lose consciousness. Hyperglycemia may also cause a loss of consciousness, although not as sudden as that caused by low blood sugar.

KEY POINT

Adult-onset diabetes, diagnosed or undiagnosed, can lead to syncope. Assess the patient's blood sugar to determine their blood glucose level.

Patients with a history of COPD may become hypoxic and lose consciousness due to decreased oxygenation of the brain. Some patients will not know they have COPD since they have not been to the doctor in years. Inquiring about a history of smoking will give a hint as to the possibility of lung disease.

The prehospital care provider should consider the difference between syncope and vertigo. Vertigo has often been confused with syncope, and the term is often improperly used. Vertigo is defined as the sense of rotation or movement of the person or their surroundings. An inner-ear infection or a problem affecting a part of central nervous system commonly causes vertigo. As an example of vertigo, consider a person complaining of "the room spinning" after consuming a large quantity of an alcoholic beverage.

A description of the event can give clues to the cause of the syncope. The patient should be asked to describe the syncopal episode including any precipitating factors: What was the patient doing just prior to and after the event? For example, a patient who describes a sudden loss of consciousness without feeling dizzy might have a cardiac rhythm disturbance such as a heart block. If the patient describes feeling dizzy without losing consciousness or dizziness just prior to syncope, the cause could be attributed to bradycardia or tachycardia. A tachycardia associated with a dizzy spell is often accompanied by palpitations.

> ### KEY POINT
>
> Have the patient describe the syncopal event. The associated signs and symptoms can give clues to the nature of the problem.

An older adult who complains of the sudden onset of respiratory distress accompanied by chest pain could be suffering from a pulmonary embolism, pneumothorax, or myocardial infarction. A detailed history of the patient's chief complaint may rule out one or more of the causes of the syncopal episode.

Patients who complain of dizziness or syncope while shaving, wearing a necktie, or while turning their head could have an overly sensitive pressure receptor (carotid sinus) in the neck. When this receptor is stimulated, the immediate response is a significant drop in the patient's heart rate and a decrease in cardiac output resulting in syncope or near-syncope.

Ask the patient if the episode was associated with urination, defecation, swallowing, or coughing. Patients with a chronic lung disease have an accompanying lower venous return to the heart and an associated decreased blood flow out of the heart. When they cough vigorously, increased pressure in the neck and chest drops the heart rate and blood pressure, leading to syncope. Similar mechanisms may be responsible for syncope associated with urination, defecation, and swallowing.

In addition to asking about physical functions that could be associated with the episode, the prehospital care provider should inquire about any significant emotional stress that may have triggered the loss of consciousness. Vasovagal syncope (simple fainting) is the sudden loss of consciousness that happens after a particularly stressful event. With vasovagal syncope, the blood vessels in the muscles dilate, reducing blood return to the heart and lowering blood pressure. Additionally, the vagus nerve to the heart is powerfully stimulated, causing a significant drop in heart rate. The end result is an instant drop in blood flow to the brain accompanied by a sudden loss of consciousness.

If the elderly patient states that they passed out when lifting something heavy or when performing some other physically exerting activity, the syncope could be attributed to a narrowing of the aorta, as in aortic stenosis, which restricts the amount of blood leaving the heart.

Finally, ask any onlookers about any muscle rigidity or jerking movements the patient may have displayed while unconscious. Muscle stiffness, such as that seen in the tonic phase of a seizure, and rhythmic jerking, such as that seen in the clonic stage of epilepsy, may indicate a seizure-related loss of consciousness.

Patient assessment should include a thorough examination of the elderly patient, including vital signs and a head-to-toe physical examination. The patient's vital signs can often give information about the cause of the syncope. The patient's blood pressure may be low (hypotension), leading to inadequate blood flow to the brain and syncope, or the blood pressure may be extremely high, hinting at the possibility of a TIA or stroke. A blood pressure that has a small difference between systolic and diastolic pressures (generally less than 30 mm HG) can indicate low blood volume or the early stages of shock. Finally, the blood pressure may significantly change with the patient's position. Orthostatic hypotension or a positive tilt test is present when the systolic blood pressure drops significantly when the patient is moved from a supine to a sitting position. In orthostatic hypotension, the blood pressure usually drops 25 to 30 mm Hg, however, the patient may become symptomatic with smaller drops in systolic blood pressure. In contrast, the elderly patient may exhibit a 40-point or more drop in systolic blood pressure and still be free of symptoms. Orthostatic hypotension can be caused by dehydration, blood loss, a weakened or ineffective blood pressure regulating system, medications that dilate blood vessels (e.g., nitrates) or slow the heart rate (e.g., calcium channel blockers) or lessen the heart's force of contraction (e.g., beta blockers). Frequently, the patient with orthostatic hypotension caused by dehydration or medication use will have rehydrated or overcome the effects of the medication prior to the arrival of the ambulance. Thus, the patient appears normal and reproducing the signs and symptoms of orthostatic hypotension may be nearly impossible.

On physical examination, any deformities of the body noted on palpation should be recorded on the patient care report and relayed to the emergency department physician. Skin turgor should be tested to determine adequacy of hydration. Keep in mind that skin turgor assessment in the elderly should not be done using the back of the hand. Rather, gently tent the skin on the cheek or abdomen and assess the elasticity of the tissues. Delayed skin turgor can indicate low fluid volume and dehydration.

The patient's cardiac rhythm should be monitored to check for any rhythm disturbances that could be related to the syncope. Sinus arrest, atrial fibrillation with a slow ventricular response, high-degree atrioventricular (AV) block, and supra- and ventricular tachycardias could contribute to the patient's loss of consciousness by impairing cardiac output.

Assess the patient's blood sugar and oxygenation. Any quick blood sugar measurement can help identify low or high blood sugar as the precipitating event. A pulse oximeter can identify hypoxia as the cause of syncope.

Using a stethoscope, listen to the patient's breath sounds to ascertain ventilation of the lungs. Also listen to the patient's carotid arteries to detect a bruit. A bruit is caused by the turbulence of blood as it passes through a narrowed artery. The narrowing could be caused by atherosclerosis or arteriosclerosis that may have decreased blood flow to the brain, causing the syncope. Document and report your findings to the emergency department physician.

Treatment of syncope begins with identifying and eliminating or treating the cause. For example, identifying and treating any abnormal cardiac rhythms such as bradycardia will treat the transient loss of consciousness. For tachydysrhythmias, finding and correcting the underlying cause will take care of the rapid heart rate. For example, a tachycardia caused by hypovolemic shock will disappear when shock is treated and corrected.

KEY POINT

Treatment of syncope begins with identifying and eliminating or treating the cause. Occasionally, probing questions are needed to clarify the etiology of the syncope.

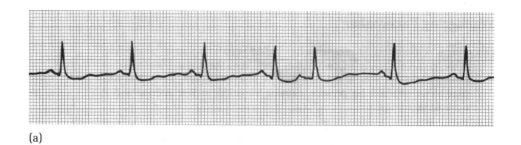

(a)

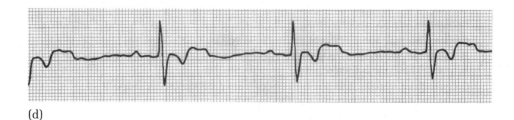

(b)

(c)

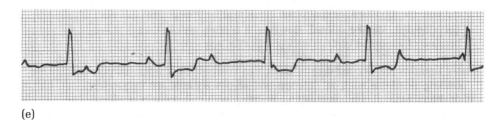

(d)

(e)

• FIGURE 8-8

Abnormal cardiac rhythms (a) premature atrial contraction (b) atrial fibrillation (c) pre-mature ventricular contractions (d) second degree AV block-Type II (e) third degree AV block.

Source: Courtesy Brady *Paramedic Emergency Care*, pp. 640–662.

In prehospital care, prehospital care providers are limited in their scope of practice. Based on the list of causes of syncope presented previously, the prehospital care provider may be able to treat some of the causes.

HEAD—Factors Related to the Central Nervous System

H	Hypoglycemia or hypoxia	Administer dextrose/administer oxygen
E	Epilepsy	Treated per protocol for seizures
A	Anxiety	Treated by emotional support, oxygen
D	Dysfunction of the brain stem	Treated by physicians

HEART—Factors Related to the Heart

H	Heart attack	Treated per protocol for AMI
E	Embolism such as pulmonary embolism	Treated per respiratory distress protocol
A	Aortic stenosis (in the elderly)	Treated by physicians
R	Rhythm disturbance	Treated per dysrhythmia protocol
T	Tachycardias, including ventricular and supraventricular tachycardia	Treated per appropriate dysrhythmia protocol

VESSELS—Factors Related to the Blood Vessels

V	Vasovagal syncope (common fainting)	Treated per protocol for simple fainting
E	Ectopic pregnancy (unlikely in elderly, but reminds of hypovolemia)	Treat for shock
S	Situational factors such as urination, defecation, and cough syncope	Treat effects per protocol, follow-up in ED
S	Subclavian steal	Treated by physicians
E	Ears, nose, and throat	Treated by physicians
L	Low SVR as seen in diabetic neuropathy	Treated by physicians
S	Sensitive carotid sinus	Loosen tight collars, physician follow-up

FEVER

Occasionally, EMS will be called to care for an elderly patient whose chief complaint consists of feeling lousy and having a fever that will not go away. Although most of these types of calls are not medical emergencies, some fevers of unknown origin (FUO) can signal severe, if not life-threatening conditions. The most significant aspect of fever in the elderly is one that relapses or does not diminish or abate after a prolonged period of time. There are many causes for fever in the elderly. A summary of those causes is presented in the following list.

Causes of Fever in the Elderly

Cancer
Infections
    Occult
    Viral
    Bacterial

Medications
Collagen vascular diseases
Recurrent pulmonary emboli
Dissecting aortic aneurysm

KEY POINT

A fever in the elderly patient is not necessarily benign—it could indicate a life-threatening condition.

Since the older adult's ability to generate heat decreases with age, the presence of a fever could herald a serious situation. Fever in children and young adults can be caused by conditions such as inflammatory bowel disease, hepatitis, lupus erythematosus and other diseases, however, these are rarely the reason for FUO in the elderly. With advancing age and decreased muscle mass and metabolism, the older adult does not produce significant amounts of heat in response to injury or illness. Thus, finding a fever in the geriatric patient can signify a serious condition and should not be taken lightly or sloughed off as a cold or the flu.

A common cause of unexplained fever in the elderly is cancer or neoplasms. Hodgkin's disease and non-Hodgkin's lymphoma are two conditions that have an associated high incidence of fever, especially in the older patient. Additionally, cancer of the kidney can produce a fever along with its typical signs and symptoms such as flank pain and blood in the urine. Liver cancer as well as cancer of the pancreas and gastrointestinal system often produce fevers. Liver cancer or cancer that has spread to the liver can produce fever, night sweats, and other symptoms that could be mistaken as an infection. Finally, a tumor of the heart, a cardiac myxoma, can produce a fever along with fatigue, weight loss, dyspnea, and peripheral edema. Initially, these findings could be interpreted as congestive heart failure.

Infections also cause fever in the elderly. Some of these infections are occult and not easily identified. Some of the occult infections include abdominal abscesses, including those in the gastrointestinal tract, liver, or kidney. A patient with a liver abscess may not have the typical jaundice or right-upper quadrant abdominal pain, causing medical personnel to overlook the possibility of a liver infection. Additionally, occult abdominal infections in the elderly may not present with abdominal pain, tenderness, or a palpable abdominal mass. One elderly man with peritonitis had a minimal fever, and, although the abdomen was rigid, he did not have abdominal tenderness or pain. Occasionally, a patient who has received a graft or prosthesis develops a postoperative infection at the graft or prosthesis site that may not be evident prior to the patient's discharge from the hospital. While the surgical site may not show any evidence of infection, internal pain and tenderness along with fever may be the only presenting signs or symptoms of an infection.

KEY POINT

Beware the hidden infection.

Another occult infection is tuberculosis. The typical tuberculosis that causes fever is miliary tuberculosis. This type of tuberculosis is characterized by small tubercles that form throughout the body as a result of the spread of the bacteria to various organs. In contrast to the expected findings of tuberculosis, the signs and symptoms of miliary tuberculosis are nonspecific. The patient's chief complaint includes fatigue, fever, weight loss, cough, altered mental status, and abdominal pain. Often, a chest X-ray will be interpreted as normal.

Finally, bacterial endocarditis can be an overlooked infection in the elderly. Patients with a subacute condition may complain of mild muscle aches or backaches. Other symptoms of bacterial endocarditis include fever, chills, headache, sweats, loss of appetite, and weight loss—all of which can be mistaken for the flu. The patient may have a heart murmur, however, a murmur could be normal for that patient. Additionally, with subacute bacterial endocarditis, the patient may show neurological signs such as hemiplegia, difficulty speaking, or seizures that may also lead the prehospital care provider away from suspecting the infection. A comprehensive work-up at the emergency department is appropriate to rule out occult infections in the elderly.

Other infections include viral and bacterial infections that are common in adults of all ages. The influenza virus affects scores of seniors each year. Although complications of the flu are uncommon in younger adults, the elderly can develop pneumonia that can lead to respiratory failure. Although annual flu shots are available, they will not totally protect a person from the flu. However, those who receive a flu shot and still contract influenza will generally develop a milder form of the disease.

Bacterial infections can develop more readily in the older adult, especially if their defenses are weakened. Superficial or skin infections can develop in patients with diabetes since impaired circulation will decrease the inflammatory response to the invading bacteria. Food poisoning, with its associated vomiting and diarrhea, could put the older adult at an increased risk for dehydration and electrolyte imbalance due to their decreased body mass and body water.

EMS personnel should be acutely aware of nosocomial infections that are transmitted between patients by healthcare workers. For example, MRSA and VRE are infections that develop in hospitalized patients or those in skilled nursing facilities. These infections are carried to other patients on the hands and clothing of caregivers. Because the older adult is more susceptible to infections, prehospital care providers should be diligent in washing their hands between patient contacts, and they should use other personal protective equipment such as gowns when moving infectious individuals.

The older adult can also develop a fever as a side effect from certain medications. These fevers can present themselves even months after the patient has started the drug therapy. In addition to the fever, the patient may complain of headache and muscle aches. The following list presents the most common medications that cause fever in the older adult.

Medications That Cause Drug-Induced Fever

Dilantin (anticonvulsant)

Quinidine (antidysrhythmia)

Tagamet (antacid)

Bactrim (antibiotic)

Septra (antibiotic)

Sulfamethoprim (antibiotic)

Atarax (antihistamine, when given IM)

KEY POINT

Some prescription medications cause fever in the older adult.

While these medications can cause a fever as long as weeks to months after the start of therapy, the fever usually goes away within 1 to 4 days after the medications are stopped. Whenever a patient reports a fever or the prehospital care provider finds a febrile patient, it is important to ask about the use of new medications.

Collagen vascular diseases such as giant cell arteritis and polyarteritis nodosa can cause fever in the elderly. While EMS rarely encounters these conditions, it is important to have some basic information about these conditions.

As the name implies, arteritis involves inflammation and swelling of the arteries. In giant cell arteritis (also called temporal arteritis), the arteries of the head and neck are involved. The patient may complain of headaches, weakness, fatigue, loss of appetite, and weight loss. Occasionally, there will be obvious swelling on the affected side of the head. Fever is also common.

In polyarteritis nodosa, a number of arteries are involved and different tissues in the body can be affected. Although the skin, kidneys, and intestines are the most likely sites of inflammation, the lungs can also be affected. With the inflammation and swelling of the arteries, blood flow to the tissues can be reduced. In addition to the signs and symptoms of giant cell arteritis, the patient with polyarteritis may also complain of abdominal pain, diarrhea, and difficulty breathing.

On occasion, patients with recurring pulmonary emboli may be febrile. These patients are usually bed-bound and have comorbid conditions that may include COPD or congestive heart failure. Patients with dissecting aortic aneurysm may also present with fever. Although this is rare, it does bring up the importance of questioning the patient about their past medical history.

In evaluating the febrile older adult, it is important to get a detailed past medical history as well as a detailed history of the present illness. Make sure to note a history of cancer and cancer therapy, as well as any medications the patient has been taking.

Be acutely aware of obvious as well as occult infections. Has the patient had a recent upper respiratory infection? Have they experienced night sweats? Have there been any changes in bowel or urinary habits? These questions and others like it are aimed at gathering information about the presence of an infection.

Oftentimes, a fever may be brushed off as merely an upper respiratory infection or other mild inflammatory disease. In the elderly, a fever can be a warning of a life-threatening condition. When in doubt about the cause of a fever, be sure to transport the patient to an emergency department for further evaluation.

The prehospital care provider should also be alert to the absence of a fever or a very low fever when the patient has a severe infection. Because of the aging process, some older adults will not have any fever although they are acutely ill.

GASTROINTESTINAL EMERGENCIES IN THE ELDERLY

The prehospital care provider may be called on to attend to an older adult with an acute abdomen. Abdominal pain with or without gastrointestinal (GI) bleeding can herald a serious, life-threatening condition. This section will discuss gastrointestinal problems the prehospital care provider may encounter when caring for the geriatric patient.

Abdominal pain can be ominous. It could mean nothing more than an episode of diarrhea, or it could signal serious internal bleeding or bowel impaction or infarct. Assessing the origin of the abdominal pain in the field is difficult at best. However, other than asking about the location of the pain, using parts of the OPQRST mnemonic for pain assessment (discussed in the chapter on patient assessment) can give clues to the etiology of the problem.

Onset	Rapid/sudden—Perforated ulcer, acute pancreatitis, dissecting aneurysm, gallstones, kidney stones
	Slow/gradual—ulcer, diverticulitis
Provoke	Eating fatty food or fruit—gallbladder disease
	Overeating—hiatal hernia
Quality	Burning pain—ulcer
	Waves of constricting pain—renal/biliary colic
	Tearing pain—aortic aneurysm
	Ache—appendicitis
	Pain progressing from colic to steady—appendicitis, strangulating intestinal obstruction, vascular problem in the gut
Radiation	Right shoulder blade—gallbladder
	Left shoulder—ruptured spleen
	Epigastric area—appendicitis
	Pubic/vaginal area—kidney
	Midback—Aortic aneurysm
Severity	Severe—perforation of hollow organ, ruptured aneurysm, arterial blockage in intestinal artery
Relief of pain	From antacids—ulcer
	From lying still—peritonitis
	Lying prone with pillow under abdomen—hiatal hernia
	Lying in a semi-Fowler's position—hiatal hernia
	Walking—biliary colic
	Nothing—kidney stone

KEY POINT

Abdominal pain in the older adult is especially ominous. A detailed history and physical examination will help identify the cause of the pain.

As there are numerous conditions that can cause abdominal pain in the elderly, it is imperative to look at a few specific diseases that may trigger the older adult's call for help. The acute abdominal conditions that this section will focus on are cholecystitis, hiatal hernia, diverticulitis, appendicitis, peritonitis, kidney stones, and gastrointestinal (GI) bleeding.

Cholecystitis is the inflammation of the gall bladder, it may also be accompanied by the formation of gall stones (cholelithiasis). Signs and symptoms of cholecystitis include indigestion, especially after eating meals that are high in fat. The patient may complain of pain in the right-upper quadrant of the abdomen that worsens when they take a deep breath. Occasionally, these patients may confuse the signs and symptoms of cholecystitis for those of an acute myocardial infarction. If gallstones completely block the bile duct, the signs and symptoms become more intense and may include unbearable pain, a fever up to 104°F, nausea, and vomiting. Treatment for an acute gallbladder attack consists of placing the patient in a position of comfort, administering oxygen if necessary, and transporting the patient to the emergency department. Definitive treatment of this condition involves surgically removing the gall bladder and any accompanying gall stones.

Signs and Symptoms of Cholecystitis

Right upper quadrant abdominal pain

Pain intensifies after high-fat meals

Pain worsens when taking a deep breath

If gallstones block bile duct, fever and nausea and vomiting are present

A hiatal hernia is a diaphragmatic hernia in which a portion of the stomach protrudes through the opening of the diaphragm into the chest cavity. Another type of esophageal hernia is the sliding hiatal hernia in which part of the stomach slides upward into the chest cavity following the normal pathway of the esophagus. The opening of the diaphragm is enlarged to allow the hernia to occur. Signs and symptoms of a hiatal hernia usually occur after a full meal and include heartburn and indigestion. A hiatal hernia can also cause abdominal and chest pain, causing the patient to suspect that they are suffering from an acute myocardial infarction. During this type of acute event, the patient may also complain of shortness of breath.

Signs and Symptoms of Hiatal Hernia

Chest and/or abdominal pain after a full meal

Heartburn and indigestion

Dyspnea

Patients usually find relief by sitting quietly with the head elevated. Some patients achieve relief in the prone position with a pillow under the abdomen.

Diverticulitis is an inflammation that occurs in the colon. A diverticulum is a sac or a pouch that develops when the mucus lining of the intestine herniates through the muscle wall of the intestine. Weakness of the muscles of the intestine caused by constipation can lead to the formation of the sac or pouch. Inflammation occurs when bacteria accumulate in the pouch and irritate the lining of the intestine. The patient often complains of cramp-like lower abdominal pain, usually in the lower-left quadrant. Rest and a bland diet may reverse the inflammation, however, in severe cases, surgery is performed to remove the inflamed tissue.

Signs and Symptoms of Diverticulitis

Left-lower quadrant abdominal pain

Cramp-like pain

History of constipation

Appendicitis is the inflammation of the appendix, which is located in the right-lower quadrant of the abdomen. If bacteria accumulate inside this tube-like structure, an infection can develop when the appendix is not allowed to drain normally. Signs and symptoms of acute appendicitis include abdominal pain that is initially felt around the navel. The umbilical pain will change to right-lower quadrant abdominal pain as the condition worsens. Rebound tenderness is typical in appendicitis. This is observed when pressure is applied to the right lower quadrant of the abdomen and suddenly released. The patient's abdominal muscles tense, and the patient bends over, guarding the area. The patient usually sits quietly, since movement can cause severe discomfort. The patient has no appetite, and may complain of nausea and vomiting. A low-grade fever is common. Since appendicitis is a surgical emergency, the patient should be promptly transported to the hospital. If the appendix ruptures, peritonitis can quickly develop.

Signs and Symptoms of Appendicitis

Umbilical pain changing to right lower quadrant abdominal pain
Rebound tenderness and guarding
Loss of appetite
Nausea and vomiting
Fever

Peritonitis is an acute inflammation of the lining of the abdomen caused by infection or irritation from the contents of a ruptured hollow organ. Internal bleeding has also been known to cause peritonitis. Signs and symptoms of peritonitis include pain over the infected or irritated site, fever, nausea, vomiting, and weakness. As the infection or irritation spreads, the abdomen becomes rigid to the touch. Since movement may aggravate the pain, the patient sits quietly. Peritonitis is also an emergent condition that is treated by antibiotics and surgery, depending on the cause.

Signs and Symptoms of Peritonitis

Abdominal pain
Rigid abdomen
Lying quietly
Fever
Nausea and vomiting
Weakness

KEY POINT

The acute abdomen is often a surgical emergency. Do not delay transport time.

Kidney stones, also known as renal calculi, are crystals formed by calcium in the kidney. Kidney stones frequently, but not always exhibit symptoms. However, kidney stones can cause inflammation and infection of the kidney, which causes pain (renal colic) and blood in the urine. When a small piece of kidney stone breaks off from a larger stone, it travels into the ureter. Since the crystal has multiple sharp points, it scrapes the lining of the ureter as it travels to the urinary bladder. This scraping causes severe flank pain and bleeding. The pain can radiate to the genitals and inner thigh. In some cases, the intense pain causes nausea and vomiting and, if an infection develops, the patient may become febrile. Patients with renal colic cannot sit or lie still. With time, the stone passes into the urinary bladder and out of the body. Occasionally, surgery or a procedure called lithotrypsy (sound waves to break up the stone) is used to treat kidney stones.

Signs and Symptoms of Kidney Stones

Severe flank pain
Restlessness
Blood in the urine
Nausea and vomiting
Fever

Frequently, older adults have episodes of acute GI bleeding. Older patients have a higher mortality rate from GI bleeding than the general population, therefore a hemorrhage from the gastrointestinal system needs to be treated promptly. Gastrointestinal bleeding can originate from two sites—the upper gastrointestinal tract and the lower gastrointestinal tract.

Common causes of upper GI bleeding include gastric and duodenal ulcers, esophageal varicies, cancers, and drug-induced bleeding. Less frequent causes of upper GI bleeding that prehospital care providers may encounter include inflammation of the stomach (gastritis) and esophageal tears (usually from protracted vomiting and retching.)

Bleeding from the GI area typically presents with vomiting of bright red blood and blood clots or coffee-ground emesis. In some cases, there may be no obvious signs of bleeding from the patient's vomitus. The signs and symptoms of shock may develop from excessive blood loss.

Blood loss from the lower GI tract is commonly caused by cancer or polyps, bleeding diverticula, hemorrhoids, colitis, and inflammatory bowel disease. Less common causes of lower GI bleeding include drugs, inflammation of the blood vessels, and ulcers of the colon. Black tarry stools are typical signs of lower GI bleeding, particularly from sites in the upper colon or small intestine. Bright red blood may be more typical of bleeding from hemorrhoids or polyps. Substantial blood loss can result in hypotension and shock.

The treatment of gastrointestinal bleeding is supportive. Administer high-flow oxygen and treat for shock. If available, initiate IV therapy with a normal saline or lactated Ringer's solution. Prompt transportation to the emergency department is required for definitive treatment of gastrointestinal bleeding.

KEY POINT

GI bleeding may not be obvious. Upper and lower GI bleeding can be life-threatening and requires prompt transportation to the emergency department.

DIABETIC EMERGENCIES

Diabetes mellitus is a life-long illness that affects millions of people. In the United States, approximately 16 million people have the disease. Unfortunately, only a little more than 10 million of these people have been diagnosed with diabetes. Over 5 million people who have the disease are unaware of their condition. Diabetes is the seventh leading cause of death in the United States.

KEY POINT

Diabetes is becoming epidemic, with an increasing number of younger people contracting the disease each year. It is a life-long disease that can have a number of serious consequences if it is not controlled.

Prehospital care providers are called to treat patients with diabetes nearly every day. Some of the calls are to treat emergency conditions brought on by the disease, whereas other calls are to care for people whose diabetes has caused other medical conditions. Prehospital care providers are familiar with diabetes from their training programs, however, it is important to review the condition with respect to the older population.

Diabetes mellitus is a general term that is applied to a group of conditions that are characterized by the body's inability to use glucose. It is primarily associated with the production and release of insulin from the beta cells of the islets of Langerhans in the pancreas. A secondary problem that is more related to adult-onset diabetes is resistance to insulin or the body's inability to use the insulin that is available.

There are two types of diabetes mellitus: Type I, or insulin-dependent diabetes mellitus (IDDM), and Type II, or non-insulin-dependent diabetes mellitus (NIDDM). Type I has also been called juvenile diabetes, whereas Type II is referred to as adult-onset diabetes. It should be noted that Type I and Type II diabetes can develop at any age. Since most older diabetics have Type II diabetes, more time will be spent on this condition.

KEY POINT

Type I diabetes is also known as insulin-dependent diabetes mellitus (IDDM). Type II diabetes is also known as non-insulin-dependent diabetes mellitus (NIDDM).

Type I and Type II Diabetes Mellitus

As a brief review, Type I diabetes (IDDM) is an autoimmune disease in which the body fails to produce insulin. Since it develops most often in childhood or in young adults, it has been called juvenile diabetes. IDDM only affects 10 to 15 percent of all known diabetic patients.

Type II diabetes (NIDDM) is found in 85 to 90 percent of all known cases. The principle underlying feature of NIDDM is a poor response of the body's tissues to the insulin that is available. It can also be caused by the body's inability to produce an adequate amount of insulin. People over 45 years of age who are obese are more likely to develop a condition known as insulin resistance—a condition in which the body cannot use or does not respond to the insulin produced by the pancreas. Insulin resistance causes the production of excess insulin, hypertension, high levels of triglycerides, low amounts of high density lipoproteins (HDL; the "good" cholesterol), and a higher incidence of atherosclerosis. These findings are also risk factors that can contribute to NIDDM. The following list summarizes the risk factors for Type II diabetes.

Risk Factors for Type II Diabetes

Over 45 years of age

Family history of diabetes

Abdominal obesity (waist >40 inches in men, >35 inches in women)

Sedentary lifestyle

Hypertension

Low HDL or high triglycerides

Women who have had gestational diabetes

Patients with Type II diabetes often show no signs or symptoms for many years. Only when the person notices something wrong do they learn of their condition. There are, however, signs and symptoms that can indicate diabetes. The following table summarizes the signs and symptoms of diabetes.

Type I Diabetes	**Type II Diabetes**
The "Polys"	Any of the signs/symptoms of Type I
• Polyuria (increased urination)	Frequent infections and delayed healing
• Polydipsia (increased thirst)	Blurred vision
• Polyphagia (increased hunger)	Delayed healing of cuts or bruises
Unusual weight loss	Altered sensations/numbness of hands and feet
Fatigue	Frequent mouth, bladder, skin infections
Ketosis/ketoacidosis	

KEY POINT

Beware of the "polys" of Type I diabetes—polyuria, polydipsia, and polyphagia.

The signs and symptoms of diabetes are associated with the pathology of the disease. As the disease progresses, the patient's blood sugar levels increase due to the body's inability to use available glucose. This creates an increase in osmotic pressure in the blood, and water from the cells (intracellular water) is moved into the circulation. The kidneys then excrete the water. Since the body excretes significant amounts of water, the patient experiences polyuria (increased urination) and polydipsia (increased thirst) to compensate for the water loss. The mechanism of polyphagia (increased hunger) is not understood, however, some theories hold that it may be the body's attempt to increase its energy supply. The fatigue is caused by ineffective glucose metabolism by the muscles.

The body's attempt to metabolize proteins and fats is incomplete and fatty acids are converted to ketones. The kidneys excrete these ketones. However, when the kidneys can no longer excrete the excess ketones, the pH of the blood begins to fall and the patient develops ketoacidosis. Ketoacidosis is potentially fatal. Ketones are highly volatile and have a sweet odor that can be noticed on the person's breath. A similar odor can be noticed from the person's urine. Not only are ketones excreted, excess glucose is also excreted by the kidneys. One hint that could be used in assessing the undiagnosed diabetic is the presence of an unusual number of ants in the bathroom, especially around the toilet. The ants are attracted to the sugar in the urine.

Patients with diabetes have poor wound healing that is thought to be caused by a decreased inflammatory response to invading microorganisms. Blood supply to the tissues is reduced due to atherosclerosis, which, in turn, reduces the number of neutrophils and macrophages available to fight a developing infection. Further, infections at the wound site are more likely since an elevated blood sugar is an excellent breeding ground for bacteria.

A visual disturbance such as blurring of vision occurs because of increased fluid inside the eye. The accumulation of fluid changes the shape of the eye and distorts the vision. Upon regulation of blood sugar levels, the visual disturbances should resolve.

Patients diagnosed with Type I diabetes will inject insulin, either on a dosing schedule or via an insulin pump. There are several types of injectable insulin available.

Types of Injectable Insulin

Humulin	Iletin I Lente
Humulin Lente	Iletin I NPH
Humulin NPH	Iletin I Regular
Humulin Regular	Iletin II Lente
Humulin Ultralente	Iletin II NPH
Humalog	Iletin II Regular

These medications are injected subcutaneously at various sites on the body. Until recently, the insulin pump was not available to seniors under Medicare guidelines. With changes in Medicare policy, older adults with hard-to-control diabetes may be eligible for the insulin pump. Therefore, prehospital care providers may increasingly encounter older patients who use the insulin pump.

Initially, mentally competent patients with Type II diabetes will control their condition through diet and exercise. They may also take any number of oral hypoglycemic (antidiabetic) medications currently available.

Oral Hypoglycemic Drugs

Tolinase (tolazamide)	Dymelor (acetohexamide)
Orinase (tolbutamide)	Amaryl (glimepride)
Glucotrol (glipizide)	Glucophage (metformin)
Diabeta. Micronase (glyburide)	Precose (acarbose)
Diabenese (chlorpropamide)	Prandin (repalinide)

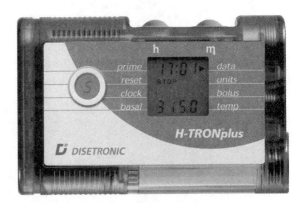

• FIGURE 8-9
Insulin pump (Disetronic) about the size of a pager.
Source: Courtesy of Disetronic.

Some of the oral hypoglycemic drugs may cause severe and potentially fatal hypoglycemia in the elderly, even when the older adult eats properly. (See chapter on pharmacology). The prehospital care provider should be aware of this potential complication and act quickly to reverse the low blood sugar. Should oral medications not control the diabetes, the patient will be prescribed insulin injections.

Control of diabetes can be especially difficult in the elderly. The following list summarizes several factors that contribute to this difficulty.

Factors Contributing to Difficult Control of Diabetes in the Elderly

Altered Senses
   Decreased vision and smell
   Decreased taste
   Decreased sense of movement/position
Difficulties preparing and consuming food
   Tremors
   Arthritis
   Altered GI function/absorption
Decreased recognition of hunger
Decreased recognition of thirst

Decreased exercise
Medications and drugs
   Diuretics
   Alcohol abuse
Psychosocial problems
   Grief/bereavement
   Depression
Poor dietary habits
Living alone
Poverty

Diabetic Emergencies

There are two primary conditions that prehospital care providers will encounter in a prehospital setting. These conditions are insulin shock and diabetic ketoacidosis (diabetic coma). Both of these conditions can be life-threatening, however, insulin shock is more rapid and can become life-threatening more quickly. The following table summarizes the clinical findings for each condition based on diagnostic signs and the patient's symptoms.

Signs and Symptoms of Insulin Shock and Diabetic Ketoacidosis

Diagnostic Sign/Symptom	Insulin Shock	Diabetic Ketoacidosis
Breathing	Normal	Deep, rapid, air hunger
Breath odor	Normal	Fruity, acetone odor
Pulse	Rapid, thready	Rapid, bounding
Skin color	Pale	Flushed
Skin temperature	Cool	Warm
Skin condition	Moist, sweaty	Dry
Pupils	Dilated	Normal
Level of consciousness	Altered	Altered
Appetite	Hungry	Hungry
Nausea/vomiting	Delayed	Delayed
Irritability	Likely	Possible
Abdominal pain	Absent	Likely

A third emergency associated with diabetes is hyperosmolar nonketotic coma. It differs from diabetic ketoacidoisis in that no acidosis is associated with this emergency. It is characterized by a severe deficiency of insulin. The small amount of available insulin produced by the pancreas may lower the ketones or fatty acids formed in the body. However, the patient's blood sugar is quite high, often above 800 mg/dL. The signs and symptoms including altered consciousness, severe dehydration, and seizures may persist for several days to weeks before the patient seeks medical help. This allows the electrolyte imbalance, dehydration, and hyperglycemia to become severe.

KEY POINT

There are three diabetic emergencies in the older adult: diabetic ketoacidosis, insulin shock, and hyperosmolar nonketotic coma.

Treatment for the older adult in diabetic crisis is the same as for a younger adult. With either insulin shock or diabetic ketoacidosis, the prehospital care provider monitors the patient's airway and vital signs, and, if appropriate, administers sugar. Giving sugar to a patient with either condition is permissible since, even in the hyperglycemic patient, sugar will not harm the patient in the short run. However, if it is obvious that the patient is hyperglycemic, sugar-containing products or solutions should not be administered.

Glucose can be administered orally if the patient is fully alert and oriented or by placing a glucose gel such as Insta-Glucose between the patient's cheek and gum. If available, IV dextrose (D50W) can be administered. With insulin shock, the response is a rapid return to full consciousness. Patients with diabetic ketoacidosis will not respond to the administration of glucose or dextrose.

Complications of Diabetes

Prehospital care providers frequently encounter patients with complications from uncontrolled diabetes. These complications include atherosclerosis with an increased risk of cardiovascular and cerebrovascular disease, diabetic neuropathies, diabetic retinopathy, and end-stage renal disease. Cardiovascular complications caused by narrowing of the arteries lead to a higher incidence of heart attack and stroke, both of which are discussed elsewhere in this chapter. End-stage renal disease is discussed in a separate chapter on the condition. The two other complications of diabetes that may impact on an older adult's quality of life, diabetic neuropathy and diabetic retinopathy, will be discussed in more detail here.

As the term implies, diabetic neuropathy is deterioration of the peripheral nervous system caused by diabetes. It is seen in approximately 60 percent of the patients with diabetes, however, many of these patients have no symptoms of neuropathy. It is more common in diabetic patients who are smokers.

Initially, the peripheral nerves of the legs are affected. Eventually, the condition may be spread over the entire body and affect many or all of the major organ systems. The condition affects the autonomic nervous system as well as the sensory nerves.

The most common form of diabetic neuropathy is peripheral neuropathy that primarily affects the nerves of the extremities. The legs and feet are especially prone to this complication. Symptoms of peripheral diabetic neuropathy include:

- Numbness or loss of sensation to pain
- Loss of sensation to temperature
- Sharp pain and cramps
- Heightened sensitivity to touch
- Decreased balance and coordination that alters gait

A major comorbidity with diabetic neuropathy is an increased risk of infection. Due to circulatory changes and the absence of pain, infections can be overlooked or not recognized and allowed to invade the body. In some severe infections that involve the deeper muscles and bone, amputation may be required as treatment of the infection. Additionally, if the patient cannot sense temperature, burn injuries such as scalds can occur more easily. Prehospital care providers should thoroughly assess the older adult diabetic for infections as well as trauma to the extremities.

If diabetic neuropathy involves the autonomic nervous system, the major organs can be affected. These organ systems include the cardiovascular system, gastrointestinal system, genitourinary system, and sweat glands of the skin.

Diabetic neuropathy affects the cardiovascular system in several ways. It can interfere with the body's ability to sense and respond to changes in blood pressure. For example, a patient may experience lightheadedness or syncope when they change from a supine to a sitting position (orthostatic hypotension). Thus, the older diabetic is at an increased risk for falls and injury, since diabetic neuropathy can also change the patient's perception of pain, and the patient might not experience chest pain or discomfort caused by angina pectoris or an acute myocardial infarction. The "silent heart attack" is more common in the diabetic population.

The gastrointestinal system is affected by changes in digestion. The stomach may be slower to empty and the patient may experience increased nausea and vomiting, loss of appetite, or a bloated sensation. Because the stomach does not move the food into the small intestine as rapidly or the patient simply does not eat, blood sugar levels may show wide swings, and the patient may range from hyperglycemia to hypoglycemia. If the esophagus is involved, the nerves of swallowing may be impaired. Nerve impairment in the intestines can lead to constipation or diarrhea as well as weight loss.

Diabetic neuropathy affecting the autonomic nerves in the genitourinary system can cause urinary retention that can lead to delirium and an increased risk of urinary tract infection. Urinary incontinence is also a problem associated with diabetic neuropathy since the patient may not be able to sense a full bladder or control when the bladder empties. Sexual function is also affected. Sexual response, but not sex drive, is decreased in both men and women. Men with diabetic neuropathy may become impotent.

Diabetic neuropathy can also affect the body's ability to sweat. The nerve damage associated with diabetic neuropathy can reduce sweating and impair the body's ability to control temperature. Occasionally, the patient may develop night sweats or sweat while eating.

Diabetic neuropathy can suddenly affect specific nerves. This typically happens in the trunk, head, or lower extremities. This focal neuropathy can cause:

- Thigh pain, usually in the front of the leg
- Pain in the lower back and the pelvic area
- Chest pain that can be mistaken for heart attack or angina
- Pain or achiness behind the eye
- Lack of ability to focus or double vision
- Bell's palsy (paralysis on one side of the face)
- Diminished hearing

Prehospital care providers should be aware of focal neuropathies, since patients experiencing chest pain may call 9-1-1 thinking that they are suffering from a heart-related problem. Or, the patient could experience Bell's palsy and think that they are having a stroke.

Another complication of diabetes that prehospital care providers should be aware of is diabetic retinopathy. While prehospital care providers will not be called on specifically for this disorder, they may need to alter their patient assessment techniques to accommodate patients with the decreased vision associated with this medical condition.

Diabetic retinopathy occurs when diabetes damages the small blood vessels that provide blood to the retina. In one form of diabetic retinopathy, retinal veins dilate and form small aneurysms that can rupture and leak blood that can cause edema of the retina. The edema can be in the peripheral vision areas, and vision changes may or may not be noticed by the patient. If the edema forms around the central part of the retina (macula), vision impairment can be significant. The central vision loss is illustrated in the following photograph.

In another type of diabetic retinopathy, new blood vessels develop around the optic disc (optic nerve). These new vessels may rupture and leak blood into the rear chamber of the eye. The new blood vessels as well as fibrous tissue that may develop, may pull on the retina and cause retinal detachment. With retinal detachment, the patient experiences loss of vision. Regardless of the type of diabetic retinopathy, the patient can experience low vision, which may impact on their quality of life and the ability to be self-sufficient. The prehospital care provider may need to alter their patient assessment and treatment techniques to accommodate for the low vision.

KEY POINT

Renal failure, diabetic retinopathy, and diabetic neuropathy are complications of uncontrolled diabetes.

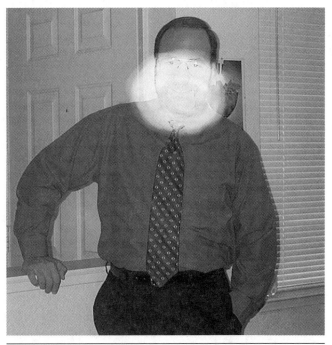

• FIGURE 8-10
Central vision loss can occur as a result of uncontrolled diabetes. Note the loss of a portion of the visual field.

Prehospital care of the older adult in a diabetic crisis is the same as for a younger adult. Establishing and maintaining a patent airway may include basic and advanced airway skills depending on the severity of the patient's condition.

HEAT AND COLD EMERGENCIES

Every summer, the news media present numerous stories about heat waves and deaths associated with those heat waves. Most of those affected by the extremes in temperature and humidity are older adults who are unable to accommodate for the high ambient temperature. However, high temperatures and humidity are not required to cause heat-related illness in the elderly. The body produces heat at all times and, depending on the level of activity, the amount of heat generated will range from 80–90 kcal (kilocalories) per hour at rest to over 900 kcal/hour with strenuous exertion. (A calorie is defined as the amount of heat required to raise 1 gram (g) of water 1 degree Celsius.) The following chart illustrates the amount of heat a person can generate at varying levels of activity. If a person is in the sun, an additional 150 kcal/hour is added to the base amount of heat generated by the body.

Heat Generation at Various Levels of Exertion

At rest	80–90 kcal/hour
Moderate exertion	300 kcal/hour
Strenuous exercise	Up to 900 kcal/hour
Being in the sun	Add 150 kcal/hour

Heat-related illness can affect older adults more easily than younger adults. The senior's ability to compensate for heat is diminished due to age-related factors such as decreased sweating abilities, decreased circulation to the skin, and a decrease in lung volume.

KEY POINT

With increasing activity, the body generates additional heat. Being in the sun adds significantly to heat production.

To dissipate heat, the body resorts to one or more physical functions. First, the body's heat regulating mechanism must be functioning properly. Heat regulation is based in the hypothalamus, which can be thought of as the body's thermostat. Its ability to regulate body temperature is contingent upon its ability to receive input from the heat sensors in the skin and organs, its ability to sense temperature changes directly from the blood, and its ability to coordinate the mechanisms to gain or eliminate heat. Because of the aging process, these mechanisms are often diminished, making the older adult more susceptible to heat-related emergencies. For some older adults, the ambient temperature has to change by more than 10°F for them to notice any change. Along with increasing age, illness or other factors such as medications can affect the body's ability to regulate heat. The following list highlights factors that predispose the older adult to heat-related illness.

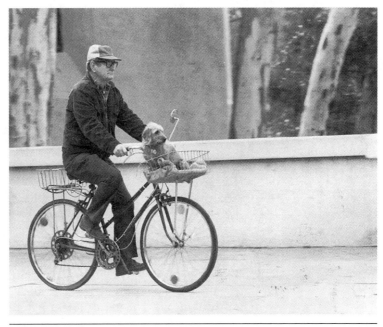

• FIGURE 8-11
Physical activity increases body heat.
Source: Courtesy of *Aging,* a magazine of the Administration on Aging.

Risk Factors for Heat-Related Illness

Lack of acclimatization
Reduced salt and water intake
Inability to tolerate hot climates
Infection
Obesity
Cardiovascular disease
Hyperthyroidism
Diabetes
Abuse of alcohol
Poor nutrition
Impaired sweat production
Problems controlling blood pressure and heart rate
Schizophrenia
Parkinson's disease
Addison's disease
Medications
    Diuretics
    Anticholinergics: Bentyl (antispasmodic), Robinul (ulcer),
    Scopolamine (motion sickness)
Phenothiazines
Antidepressants: tricyclic antidepressants and MAO inhibitors
Antihistamines
Thyroid hormones
Beta blockers: Atenolol, Propranolol, Labetolol, Corgard
Methyldopa (blood pressure control)
Aspirin (in higher doses)

Heat Loss Mechanisms

When exposed to elevated temperatures or physical exertion, the body may gain heat. With heat gain, the hypothalamus stimulates the reflexes of the body to dilate the blood vessels and begin sweating. The body attempts to eliminate the additional heat using one or more of the following five methods: Evaporation, conduction, convection, radiation, and increased rate and depth of ventilation. In evaporation, the body sweats and releases heat as the perspiration evaporates. As much as 20 percent of the body's heat is dispersed in this manner. A contributing factor to the body's ability to disperse heat through sweating is the relative humidity of the air. The more moisture in the air, the less heat the body loses through sweating since the sweat does not evaporate. The heat index is a tool that shows the effects of increasing humidity and temperature as they pertain to their combined effects on the body. The following chart shows the Heat Index.

Heat Index*

Air Temperature Relative humidity (%)	70°	75°	80°	85°	90°	95°	100°	105°	110°	115°	120°
					Apparent Temperature						
0	64	69	73	78	83	87	91	95	99	103	107
10	65	70	75	80	85	90	95	100	105	111	116
20	66	72	77	82	87	93	99	105	112	120	130
30	67	73	78	84	90	96	194	113	123	135	148
40	68	74	79	86	93	101	110	122	137	151	
50	69	75	81	88	96	107	120	135	150		
60	70	76	82	90	100	114	132	149			
70	70	77	85	93	106	124	144				
80	71	78	86	97	113	136	157				
90	71	79	88	102	122	150	170				
100	72	80	91	108	133	166					

*All temperatures are in °F.

In conduction, heat is transferred to another surface or substance. For example, when a person is immersed in cool water such as a bath or pool, body heat is rapidly dispersed into the cooler water. The colder the surface or substance, the faster the cooling effect on the body. In contrast, exposure to overly warm water can induce a heat illness. Consider a hot tub that has been heated to more than 105°F. When a person immerses him or herself in the hot water, the heat is conducted into the body, raising the core temperature. Without an adequate defense or mechanism to lower the increasing body temperature, heat exhaustion or heat stroke can quickly develop.

The body also eliminates heat through convection. When a breeze blows across the body, it removes the heat and reduces the body's temperature. Some studies have shown that to effectively cool a body by convection, the breeze or wind should be at least 16 to 18 mph.

The body also gives off heat from the skin into the environment through radiation, although this mechanism is not very effective.

Finally, the respiratory system gives off heat each time a person breathes. When the pulmonary capillaries dilate, heat is transferred into the air inside the alveoli, which is then exhaled out of the body.

KEY POINT

Heat loss mechanisms include evaporation, conduction, convection, radiation, and breathing. Any or all of these mechanisms can be impaired in the older adult.

The older adult's response to high temperatures is based on changes in physiology with aging. In some patients, a decreased ability to sweat reduces the body's effectiveness in eliminating heat gain. In other patients, excessive sweating and vasodilation leads to a drop in arterial blood pressure. When the blood pressure falls, the reflex response is to constrict peripheral blood vessels. If this occurs, blood flow to the skin is reduced, decreasing the heat-loss mechanism through the skin. The net effect would be to increase the core body temperature, further raising the risk of a heat-related illness.

Heat-Related Emergencies

There are four heat-related emergencies the prehospital care provider may be called to assess and treat. These conditions include heat edema, heat cramps, heat exhaustion, and heat stroke.

Heat edema is seen in individuals who are not acclimatized to heat and humidity. The body responds to heat by retaining sodium and water. The result is peripheral edema, typically in the lower extremities. This edema is limited to the legs, and there are no other indications of fluid overload such as increased blood pressure or pulmonary edema. The patient has a history of heat exposure and complains of unusual swelling of their feet and ankles. Treatment is minimal—eliminate the heat, allow the body to cool normally, and elevate the legs. There is no need for diuretics. With gradual acclimatization, heat edema will be less of a problem.

Heat cramps occur when people in a hot environment replace lost fluids but do not replace lost body salt. The sodium and potassium depletion causes skeletal muscle cramping, which has been described as intermittent, intense, and very painful. The abdominal muscles are those that are typically involved. Heat cramps develop several minutes to hours after exposure to the heat, thus there may be no obvious indication as to the nature of the patient's problem. Careful assessment and questioning can elicit information pertaining to heat exposure.

Like heat edema, heat cramps are easily treated. Since there may be no indication of heat exposure, it may not be necessary to remove the heat source. The best form of treatment for heat cramps is to increase the dietary consumption of salt and potassium. The oral administration of an electrolyte solution such as Gatorade may be effective. If a commercially available electrolyte solution is not available, mix a half-teaspoon of salt in a glass of water and instruct the patient to sip the solution. Bananas are an effective source of potassium. The use of salt tablets is not advisable. Salt tablets can cause gastric irritation as well as fluid shifts into the bowel. Thus, water replacement into the body is not assured.

Heat exhaustion is the next level of heat-related illness. It can be caused by water depletion, salt depletion, or depletion of both water and salt. Typically, heat exhaustion caused by salt depletion is found in younger adults, whereas heat exhaustion caused by water depletion is more common in the elderly. The primary reason for water-depletion heat exhaustion is due to restricted water intake, possibly because of limited mobility, a reduced sense of thirst, or other, similar reasons. EMS will most often see water-depletion heat exhaustion during prolonged heat waves. The signs and symptoms of both water-depletion and salt-depletion heat exhaustion are listed in the following table.

Signs and Symptoms of Heat Exhaustion

Salt-Depletion Heat Exhaustion	Water-Depletion Heat Exhaustion
Body temperature normal or low	Body temperature elevated (up to 103°F)
Fatigue	Intense thirst
Weakness	Weakness
Nausea and vomiting	Anxiety or restlessness
Diarrhea	Confusion/impaired judgment
Loss of appetite	Tingling sensations in hands/feet
Headache	Increased skin turgor
Giddiness	Abnormal behavior (psychotic-like)
Muscle cramps	Lack of muscle coordination
Pale, moist skin	Muscular tetany
Weak, rapid pulse	Weak, rapid pulse
Hypotension	Altered level of consciousness
Altered mental states	Loss of consciousness
Loss of consciousness	May progress to heat stroke

Although it appears that water-depletion heat exhaustion is similar to heat stroke, there is one major difference—body temperature. The onset of heat stroke begins with a body temperature of 105°F and climbs. However, there are times when differentiating between water-depleted heat exhaustion and heat stroke is difficult.

Treatment for heat exhaustion includes removing the patient from the environment and allowing them to cool. Applying cool, moist towels on the forehead, back of the neck, armpits, groin, and abdomen is appropriate. Since the older patient may have an adequate amount of salt in their system, adding an electrolyte solution may not be best in the prehospital setting. However, administering fluids orally or intravenously (D5W or normal saline) to begin rehydration would be appropriate. Older adults should be transported to the emergency department for further evaluation. Having the older adult drink a glass of salted water and instructing them to remain out of the heat, may imperil the patient's life. Allowing the patient to return to or remain in the hot environment could easily precipitate heat stroke.

Heat stroke is the most severe of the heat-related illnesses and has two categories, classic and exertional. Exertional heat stroke, typically seen in younger patients, occurs when the body's ability to disseminate heat does not keep up with heat gain. The patient's muscular exertion in a hot environment outpaces their ability to get rid of the extra heat. These patients are often sweating and have skin that is cool to the touch. These findings often cover an increased core temperature.

The older adult is more likely to suffer classic heat stroke. Classic heat stroke is seen in epidemic proportions in areas hit by prolonged heat waves. Patients with existing medical problems or those taking medications that dispose them to heat illness are more likely to suffer heat stroke. The signs and symptoms associated with heat stroke are presented in the following list.

Signs and Symptoms of Heat Stroke

Flushed skin

Hot, dry skin

Elevated body temperature (>105°F)

Temperature ≥103°F accompanied by altered mental status

Rapid, bounding pulse

Dilated pupils

Increased rate and depth of breathing initially, then apnea

Altered mental states, including psychotic-like behavior

Seizures

Coma

Death

Patients with heat stroke will have significant alterations of their mental status. Initially, patients will be confused, but can quickly become comatose. Once cooling begins, the prehospital care provider can expect chills, shivering, and seizures as the core temperature drops. The patient may also display nuchal rigidity as well as various pupil abnormalities. The patient's level of consciousness generally improves quickly, and the body temperature cools. However, patients who remain comatose even after cooling often have a poorer prognosis.

Complications of heat stroke include peripheral neuropathy, ataxia, nystagmus, dementia, and occasionally, stroke-like signs. Liver function impairment and renal failure are complications associated with exertional heat stroke, as is disseminated intravascular coagulation (a blood clotting disorder).

Treatment for heat stroke includes rapid cooling and prompt transportation to an emergency department. If a core thermometer is available, monitor the patient's temperature and attempt to cool the patient to 102°F. As always, maintaining a patent airway and ventilation with or without mechanical assistance (intubation) are essential. If an airway is secure, administer high-flow oxygen. Since the older adult's heat stroke may be associated with water depletion, establish two IVs with either lactated Ringers solution or saline. The patient's ECG should be monitored continuously.

Begin cooling the patient by removing them from the heat source, removing as many of the patient's clothes as possible and wrapping the patient in cool, wet towels. Be sure to change the towels frequently since heat from the patient will be conducted to the towels. Use ice packs on the forehead, the nape of the neck, chest, and abdomen, in the armpits, groin, and behind the knees. Do not cover the patient in ice or immerse them in an ice bath. Be prepared for shivering and seizures. If the patient begins to shiver, slow the cooling process slightly since shivering generates heat. When the shivering subsides, continue cooling the patient. It is important to begin the cooling process as soon as possible to prevent or minimize the complications of heat stroke.

KEY POINT

The four types of heat illness include heat edema, heat cramps, heat exhaustion, and heat stroke.

Hypothermia is also of concern in the elderly population. Hypothermia exists when the core temperature is lower than 95°F. This is considered a medical emergency. Hypothermia can occur when a person is exposed to very low temperatures or when a person with impaired heat-regulating mechanisms is exposed to slightly cooler ambient temperatures. The heat loss mechanisms that were discussed in the section on heat illness are the same mechanisms responsible for hypothermia—evaporation, conduction, convection, and radiation. While sweating is not a major contributor to hypothermia, any moisture on the skin can evaporate and lower the body's temperature. Consider, for example, the patient in shock with cool, clammy skin. The diaphoretic patient loses body heat through evaporation, and can become hypothermic depending on the ambient temperature. Thus, a general procedure of maintaining body heat for a patient in shock is a standard of care.

KEY POINT

Extremes in temperature do not have to occur to cause hypothermia in the older adult.

Patients who are immersed in cold water are at particular risk for hypothermia since the body will rapidly conduct heat into the cold water. Some experts have indicated that water does not have to be extremely cold to induce hypothermia. It has been suggested that immersion in water that is less than 95°F can slowly cause a drop in core body temperature. Hypothermia can develop quickly depending upon the water temperature. The following chart lists the average survival times for various water temperatures.

Survival Times for People Immersed in Cold Water

Water Temp. (°F)	Length of Survival
28 (i.e., salt water)	Approx. 15 minutes
32	15–30 min
40	30–90 min
50	1–4 hours
60	2–24 hours
70	3–40 hours
80	indefinitely

Patients also lose heat and become hypothermic by convection. Any wind or breeze blowing across the skin will reduce heat. Consider the wind-chill factor that the news media reports every winter. (See wind-chill factor table.) In temperature extremes, exposed flesh can freeze in mere seconds with a brisk wind. For example, at −30°F with a 30 mph wind, exposed skin can freeze in 30 seconds!

Finally, radiation can lower the body's temperature. While this process is slow in the average-aged adult, it can occur more quickly in the senior citizen.

In normal, healthy adults, hypothermia is not a common event unless there are extremes in temperature. However, older adults may be at higher risk due to

Wind Chill Chart*

Wind Speed (mph)	Temperature (°F)								
Calm	40	30	20	10	0	−10	−20	−30	−40
5	36	25	13	1	−11	−22	−34	−46	−57
10	34	21	9	−4	−16	−28	−41	−53	−66
15	32	19	6	−7	−19	−32	−45	−58	−71
20	30	17	4	−9	−22	−35	−48	−61	−74
25	29	16	3	−11	−24	−37	−51	−64	−78
30	28	15	1	−12	−24	−39	−53	−67	−80
35	28	14	0	−14	−27	−41	−55	−71	−82
40	27	13	−1	−15	−29	−43	−57	−72	−84
						Frostbite 10 min.		Frostbite 5 min.	

*All temperatures are in °F.

Source: Adapted from NOAA Wind Chill Chart effective November 1, 2001.

underlying factors that predispose them to hypothermia. The factors that can increase the chance of cold-related emergency are presented in the following list.

Factors Predisposing a Person to Hypothermia

Advancing age
Cerebrovascular disease, including tumors, stroke, and dementia
Psychosis, including schizophrenia
Hypothyroidism
Diabetes mellitus
Kidney failure
Liver failure
Malnutrition
Infections
    Tuberculosis
    Peritonitis
    Meningitis
Pancreatitis
Alcohol abuse
Medications
    Phenothiazines (Pentazine, Phenergan)
    Tricyclic antidepressants (Elavil, Triavil)
    Benzodiazepines (Valium, Librium)
    Morphine
    Reserpine
    Barbiturates (Seconal)
    Meprobamate
Congestive heart failure

When a person is exposed to a cold environment, the hypothalamus senses the cold temperature and responds with peripheral vasoconstriction. The reduced blood flow to the periphery and shunting of blood to the central circulation acts to protect the vital organs, including the brain, heart, lungs, and abdominal organs. This vasoconstriction also preserves heat by reducing heat loss through evaporation, conduction, convection, and radiation. As the core temperature drops, the body responds by generating heat through increased metabolism and shivering.

These defense mechanisms may be altered in the older adult. The older adult may not be able to easily detect a temperature change. As mentioned in the discussion of heat-related emergencies, the senior citizen's ability to recognize changes in temperature is impaired. Some patients may not recognize a temperature change until the ambient temperature has changed by at least 10°F. Aging may decrease the patient's ability to constrict their peripheral blood vessels. Additional heat loss is possible, and the core temperature is at risk for a quick drop. Aging also slows metabolism and decreases the person's ability to shiver. Thus, the older adult's ability to generate heat is severely impaired. Because of aging, decreased mobility, the absence of hunger, or the loss of appetite, the older adult may have less subcutaneous fat to act as insulation against the low temperature.

As core temperature drops, the clinical findings will change. The following list will help identify some physical signs and symptoms associated with varying core temperatures.

Mild Hypothermia (> 95°F)

Feeling cold
Shivering (begins close to 95°F)
Normal level of consciousness

Moderate Hypothermia (> 90°F)

Shivering decreases and is replaced by muscle stiffness
Mentation deteriorates and the patient may appear to be intoxicated, irrational, or confused
Simple tasks are difficult to perform

Severe Hypothermia (< 90°F)

Shivering ceases, replaced by muscle rigidity
Altered level of consciousness/coma
Bradycardia
Hypotension
Irregular cardiac rhythm
Peripheral tissues may begin to freeze
Cardiac arrest develops when core temperature is < 86°F

Specific organ systems are also affected by hypothermia. Of particular note to prehospital care providers are the cardiovascular system, central nervous system, respiratory system, and urinary system. As the core temperature continues to fall, the heart rate and cardiac rhythm will be affected. Because of its effects on the atrial and ventricular pacemakers, hypothermia will slow the heart rate and cause bradycardia. Even though the heart rate is slower, the patient's blood pressure is generally maintained because of vasoconstriction. Dysrhythmias other than bradycardia are also common. Atrial fibrillation commonly develops in hypothermic patients. Premature ventricular contractions (PVCs) are also common, and can lead to ventricular fibrillation, especially when the core temperature falls to 86°F. Finally, when the core temperature falls to nearly 80°F, the heart will stop completely.

The central nervous system is protected by hypothermia because metabolism by the brain and spinal cord decrease under cold conditions. This explains why hypothermic patients have been successfully resuscitated even after prolonged cardiopulmonary arrest. However, hypothermia does have some adverse effects on the CNS that may affect a person's ability to function. Gait and fine motor skills deteriorate with a reduction in body temperature. Altered mental states are common and, unless the hypothermia is corrected, the patient will become incoherent and eventually comatose.

The drop in core temperature affects the respiratory system. Ventilation becomes shallow and slow, causing carbon dioxide retention as well as hypoxia. The prehospital care provider should be prepared to provide assisted ventilation to the hypothermic patient. However, endotracheal intubation should be avoided as it can overstimulate the airway and precipitate ventricular fibrillation.

Hypothermic patients will often become incontinent. With peripheral vasoconstriction, there is an increased amount of blood in central circulation. The kidneys, influenced by the blood volume as well as a reduced level of antidiuretic hormone, respond by undergoing a "cold diuresis" and excrete a large amount of water. When the patient is rewarmed, they may be hypotensive due to a decrease in overall blood volume.

Prehospital treatment of hypothermia will depend on the severity of the condition. Here are a few guidelines for basic and advanced life-support treatment for the hypothermic patient. The first step in treating hypothermia is recognizing it! While that sounds simplistic, hypothermia is an underreported condition that can have deleterious long-term effects. Suspect hypothermia when assessing a patient who seems excessively sleepy or confused or one who has slow, slurred speech. Again, the ambient temperature does not have to be extremely cold to induce hypothermia in the senior citizen.

In all cases of suspected hypothermia, remove any wet garments and cover the patient with a dry blanket. Ensure adequate breathing and provide supplemental oxygen as necessary. Monitor all vital signs and, if available, monitor the patient's ECG. If a core thermometer is available, it should be used to monitor the patient's temperature.

The treatment goal in mild or early hypothermia is to rewarm the patient. Remove the patient from the cold environment and place them in a warm, dry area. The back of a heated ambulance will provide the warmth necessary to recover from a mild chill. Mild exercise (moving arms and legs) is acceptable, but only if the patient's core temperature is about 95°F. Unless contraindicated or not available, give the patient warmed, sweetened liquids to sip. Do not allow the patient to smoke or drink alcoholic beverages.

For moderate hypothermia, keep the patient still. Do not allow the patient to exercise, and remember that rough handling can trigger ventricular fibrillation. Apply warm compresses to the patient's chest, trunk, back of the neck, arm pits, and groin to facilitate warming. If available, start an IV with warmed normal saline.

Warming IV solutions can be accomplished in a couple of ways. To have warmed IV solutions available throughout the shift, place a large bottle filled with hot water into an ice chest (cooler). Place a variety of IV solutions (D5W, lactated Ringer's, and normal saline) into the cooler and seal it closed. This will warm the solutions and keep them warm for several hours. Replace the hot water as necessary to keep the solutions warm. During extremely cold months, medications can be prevented from freezing in the same manner. Another option is wrapping a hot pack around an IV solution to keep it warm during on-scene and transport time. Once the patient has been rewarmed, keep the patient warm and do not allow reexposure or reinjury. Administer warm, moist oxygen by face mask. To warm the oxygen, wrap a hot pack around the oxygen humidifier.

For severe hypothermia, handle the patient gently and do not rewarm the patient. Instead, remove any wet clothing and cover the patient with blankets to maintain their current temperature. Rewarming the patient with external heat will cause peripheral vasodilation and can result in rewarming shock. Monitor all vital signs and ECG. Provide basic and advanced life-support as appropriate. If the patient develops cardiac arrest, provide CPR. EMS personnel should continue CPR until the patient has been delivered to an emergency department where CPR and other resuscitation techniques can be continued.

The severely hypothermic patient is not likely to respond to advanced resuscitation measures such as medications and defibrillation. Thus, defibrillation is not recommended for severely hypothermic patients. Further, local protocols should determine if medications are to be administered. Although no one has developed dosing schedules, doses for cardiac medications should be reduced, since some drugs can accumulate to toxic levels due to decreased metabolism. Experts suggest that medications not be administered unless the patient's core temperature is at least 86°F.

In any case of hypothermia, the old adage is well-founded: He ain't dead 'til he's warm and dead!

SUMMARY

This chapter has presented information on the medical emergencies that older adults are likely to experience. Although many elderly patients face similar emergencies as younger adults, advancing age may compromise their responses and ability to compensate for the acute problem. For the older adult, respiratory and cardiovascular emergencies pose a significant threat. This chapter also presented information on gastrointestinal emergencies, syncope, and environmental emergencies. In reviewing the acute and chronic conditions here, it is easy to see why the older adult is such a tremendous challenge to EMS. By being familiar with medical emergencies frequently found in the older adult, the astute prehospital care provider will be able to recognize and respond to the challenges posed by the older adult in crisis.

ON THE JOB

It is a warm spring day and you are called to a park in response to a call for a "man down." Upon arrival, you find a 72-year-old man sitting on the grass near a picnic area. Some friends of his who are concerned about the man's condition are supporting him in the sitting position. According to the bystanders, the man was walking briskly after lunch when he suddenly collapsed. According to the patient, he got "weak and dizzy" before he passed out. What are the causes of syncope in the older adult? Being that it is a warm spring day, describe the contributing effects of heat and exercise on the patient's syncope. What are the treatment options for this patient?

9

Accidental Injuries

OBJECTIVES

At the end of the chapter, the reader will be able to:

1 List 10 causes of falls in elderly patients.
2 List the signs and symptoms of a compression fracture of the spine and a fractured rib.
3 State the general cause of decubitus ulcers.
4 Describe the differences among the four stages of decubitus ulcers.
5 List six criteria that put the older adult at a high-risk for burn injury.
6 List the signs, symptoms, and treatment for carbon monoxide poisoning.

FALLS

Accidents are the fifth leading cause of death in people over 65 years of age. Falls account for two-thirds of the deaths caused by accidents. Sadly, falls are common in the elderly. Statistics show that one in three people over the age of 65 suffers a fall each year. Falls have also been attributed with high mortality in the older adult. It is estimated that 50 percent of the patients who fall and are hospitalized will not be alive 1 year after the fall. The biggest reason for increased mortality after a fall is reduced mobility or immobility. For example, approximately half of the patients who could walk prior to a hip fracture were unable to walk after the injury.

The decreased mobility after a fall is referred to as postfall syndrome. The lack of activity after the fall injury can lead to stiff joints, muscle wasting from inactivity, and a further decline in mobility. Reduced mobility can lead to a higher incidence of pneumonia, hypothermia, dehydration, malnutrition, and decubitus ulcers. This cascade of problems can significantly contribute to the death of the adult even though the initial fall was seemingly minor.

The consequences of a fall are numerous. They include soft tissue injuries; fractures to the hip, femur, humerus, wrist, ribs; and, at times, a subdural hematoma. Many older adults sustain injuries from what would appear to be a minor fall—one that would be nearly inconsequential as a younger adult. As a result of these injuries, the older adult may be hospitalized and immobilized. With immobility come additional risks to the elder's health, such as pulmonary embolism and decubitus ulcers.

KEY POINT

A major complication of a fall injury is immobility.

Reasons for falling include many age-related factors, which, if monitored and corrected, can prevent the fall. Some of the age-related factors include poor posture, changes in the way the person walks, and pathological conditions that tend to decrease a person's stability while standing or walking. It is important to identify the cause of the fall to prevent overlooking a serious, underlying medical problem.

Poor posture is not just slouching. As a person ages, the proprioreceptors (brain sensors that inform the nervous system about position and movement) deteriorate. The older adult may not be able to fully determine changes in body position when going from a sitting to an upright position. Stepping forward before securing full balance could lead to a fall. With decreased muscle tone, changing positions or becoming fully upright may be difficult. If the older adult is still leaning forward while attempting to walk, an altered center of gravity could cause a fall.

KEY POINT

Poor posture can contribute to falling by putting the older adult off balance.

Many older adults do not pick up their feet as high when they walk as they did when they were younger. Older men tend to have a flexed posture and a wide gait with short steps. Women, in contrast, have a narrow gait and tend to waddle when they walk. Thus, many elderly appear to shuffle when walking. A shuffling gait may also be caused by poor eyesight and reduced depth perception.

Pre-existing conditions or medical problems that can lead to a fall include those that lead to or contribute to a person's stability on their feet. These conditions include degenerative joint disease, especially in the knee. A prior hip or femur fracture can lead to difficulty walking and loss of stability, as can a previous stroke. Patients with diabetes may have neuropathies that can result in poor sensations in the feet and legs. If a person cannot feel their feet, ankles, or lower legs, they can lose their balance and easily fall. Many elderly patients complain of pain in their feet due to a disease or deformity such as a bunion, bone spur, corn, or callus. Pain while walking can cause a person to use a gait that will ease the discomfort, which can trigger a fall. Patients with diminished vision are also at risk for falls.

It is easy to see why older adults, especially those with underlying medical conditions, are disposed to falling. However, there are a number of reasons that the elderly may suffer a fall. It is important for the prehospital care provider to ask about the cause of the fall, as it could have been the result of an acute illness that needs prompt medical attention. The following table identifies causes of falls. However, it may not be easy to identify the reason for the fall as, in some cases, the older adult may not remember the incident or there may not be any witnesses to the event. However, prehospital care providers need to query the patient to see if any underlying pathology could have contributed to the fall.

Causes of Falls

Type of Fall	Cause
Accidental fall	Slip, trip, misstep
	Spontaneous hip fracture
	Syncope
	Sudden weakness in one or both legs
	Dizziness
	Alcohol use or abuse
Medication-related fall	Antidepressants (watch for postural hypotension)
	Antihypertensive drugs (may cause hypotension)
	Antipsychotic drugs (may sedate the patient
	Diuretics (can cause hypovolemia)
Falls due to acute medical problems	Cardiac dysrhythmias
	Stroke
	TIA
	Seizures
	Brain tumor
	Subdural hematoma

In addition to querying the patient about the cause of the fall, the prehospital care provider can, if time permits, assess the patient's environment to identify hazards that could increase the risk of falling. The following table highlights environmental factors that may lead to a fall.

Lighting—too dim or too bright	Hard to reach kitchen cabinets
Hard to reach light switches	Kitchen floor waxed or wet
Loose or worn carpets	Slippery bathtub
Unstable chairs and tables	No supports around bathtub
Chairs with no armrests	Toilet too low
Furniture blocking pathways	Medicine cabinet too high
Cold room temperature	No handrails on stairs
Extension cords over rugs	Outside steps uneven
Doors sticking or hard to open	Cracked sidewalks

If a fall hazard exists, the prehospital care provider should make suggestions to repair or eliminate the hazard. If the patient is unable to make the repairs, a family member, caregiver, or landlord could be consulted about making the environment safer.

FRACTURES

As mentioned earlier, fractures can be a contributing cause of or the result of a fall. One of the major causes of fractures is osteoporosis—an excessive loss of calcium from the bones resulting in a loss of bone mass. Older adults typically sustain some form of calcium loss from their bones, however, in some cases, there is an excessive loss of calcium that can be caused by either a hormone (estrogen) deficiency, as seen in some postmenopausal women, or a calcium-poor diet. Loss of bone mass can also be caused by lack of use. When a bone is not subject to weight-bearing stress, it tends to lose bone mass. Some estimates hold that after only 6 months of immobility, up to 40 percent of the initial bone mass may be lost. Bone mass can also be lost as a result of excess amounts of endocrine hormones or the presence of some forms of cancer. Regardless of the cause of osteoporosis, the condition puts the older adult at risk of a broken bone anywhere in the body.

With the loss of bone mass, an incident that should be a minor trauma can result in a fracture. A cough, a turn, or the twisting of the upper body could cause a rib fracture. A sudden turn while standing can cause a broken hip, as can a seemingly gentle fall. Sitting down firmly can cause a compression fracture of the spine. Nontraumatic fractures, called stress fractures, can occur in the feet, the tibia, and other long bones of the body.

KEY POINT

Osteoporosis can lead to fractures, including nontraumatic fractures.

A rib fracture results in severe pain to touch and movement and often in pain on inspiration. Crepitus on inspiration may be heard with a stethoscope or felt by palpation with the hand. The treatment for a rib fracture in the elderly is the same as that for a younger adult—immobilize the injury with a sling and swathe or use a small pillow gently bound to the chest. If respiratory distress is evident, supplemental oxygen should be administered. Typically, rib fractures caused by osteoporosis do not cause displacement of the rib. Thus, the incidence of a pneumothorax, hemothorax, or flail chest is not common in osteoporotic fractures. A flail chest may occur as a result of a motor vehicle accident or other significant impact injury. Flail chest is treated the same in the elderly as in the younger adult—high-flow oxygen, immobilization of the flail segment with towels or pillow taped to the chest and, if needed, assisted ventilation using bag-valve-mask or intubation.

Signs of a Fractured Rib

Chest pain
Pain on palpation
Crepitus
Difficulty breathing
Pain on deep inspiration

Occasionally, a compression fracture of one of the vertebrae will occur either spontaneously or as the result of sitting forcefully. Most often, the vertebrae of the thoracic and lumbar spine are affected. The signs and symptoms of a compression fracture include localized pain over the fracture site that spreads around the trunk bilaterally. The pain will be especially sharp on percussion of the involved vertebrae. Because the pain may be extreme, the patient may "splint" him or herself into a position of comfort. Deep breathing, coughing, turning, moving, sitting, standing, or walking can worsen the pain. Because of the nature of the fracture, spinal cord involvement is rare.

KEY POINT

Sitting abruptly can cause a compression fracture of the spine.

Prehospital treatment of compression fractures due to osteoporosis includes transportation of the patient in a position of comfort and supplemental oxygen if breathing is inhibited due to the pain. Analgesics can be administered on the advice of the emergency department physician. Placing the patient on a long spine board may not be advisable for several reasons. First, the patient has already splinted him or herself by getting into the position of comfort. Moving the patient to a supine position may exacerbate the pain. Second, the likelihood of spinal cord involvement is minimal, therefore complete immobilization including cervical spine precautions is not warranted. Third, a history of vertebral compression fractures may have caused severe hunching of the back (kyphosis), making spinal immobilization nearly impossible. In one case, the patient's kyphosis was so severe that while in a supine position, the back of his head was 6 inches from the surface of the backboard. The patient's head, neck, and back had to be supported with pillows to facilitate transportation. An option for immobilizing the head, neck, and spine in this instance is a vacuum splint mattress such as the MDI Full Body mattress or the Ferno mattress. This device allows immobilization of the patient in any position without applying unnecessary pressure to the older adult's delicate skin.

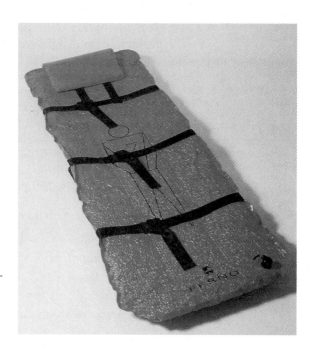

• FIGURE 9-1
Vacuum mattress splint by
Ferno.
Source: Courtesy of Ferno.

Signs and Symptoms of a Compression Fracture of the Spine

Severe pain
Pain on palpation
Pain on deep inspiration
Worsening of pain on percussion of vertebrae
Patient splints self in position of comfort

Hip fractures affect a large number of older adults each year. Estimates indicate that one in three women and one in eight men will sustain a hip fracture before death. Currently, there are over 250,000 hip fractures annually, and 12 to

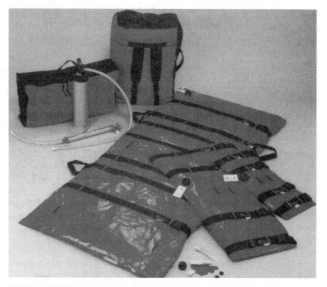

• FIGURE 9-2
MDI vacuum splint.
Source: Courtesy of Medical Devices International.

29 percent of those who suffer a hip fracture will die as a result of or complications from the injury.

With osteoporosis, a hip fracture can occur spontaneously or after a fall. Patients may have sustained the fracture while turning or twisting their lower body. The most common sites for the fracture include the proximal end of the femur and the area between the greater and lesser trochanter and head of the femur (see the following illustration).

Signs of a fractured hip include pain at the fracture site, shortening of the affected leg, and an outward rotation of the foot on the affected leg. The patient is unable to lift or move the leg and is unable to walk. Although rare, pain around the knee on the affected side may also be present. Other signs and symptoms may include swelling and discoloration at the fracture site.

Signs and Symptoms of a Fractured Hip

Pain localized around the hip

Swelling and discoloration

Pain in the knee area (rare)

Shortened leg

Outward rotation of the affected leg

Inability to lift or move the leg

Inability to walk

Prehospital care of the patient with a hip fracture includes stabilizing the leg by binding it to the other leg. Place a blanket between the legs, then apply cravats to bind the legs together. Another option is to use padded long boards along the side of the patient and along the inside of the affected leg. Tie the boards together using cravats (see below). If the situation warrants, spinal precautions can be implemented.

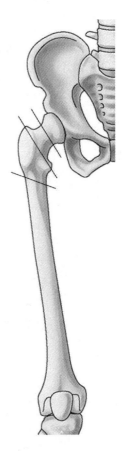

• FIGURE 9-3
Common sites for hip fractures.
Source: Courtesy Brady *MedEMT,* p. 95.

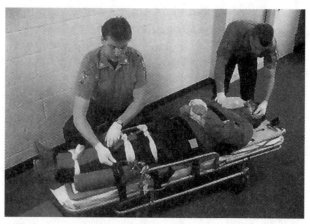

(a)

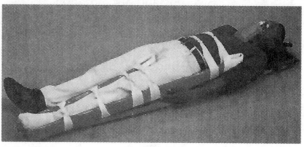

(b)

• FIGURE 9-4
(a) Immobilize hip fractures by binding the legs together or (b) using board splints.
Source: Courtesy Brady *Emergency Care* 8th ed., p. 569.

HEAD INJURY—SUBDURAL HEMATOMA

Another consequence of a fall is a subdural hematoma. This is an accumulation of blood inside the skull, under the dura mater. The dura mater is one of the meninges (membranes) covering of the brain. A subdural hematoma is typically caused by blunt head trauma. There is no associated skull fracture. The injury jostles the brain and causes veins in the head to rupture, causing blood to collect around the injury site. Blood gradually continues to accumulate and, since the skull is rigid, the collection of blood begins to put pressure on the brain. As the pressure continues to increase, the patient's condition deteriorates. The deterioration can take days to weeks to develop.

> ### KEY POINT
>
> Bleeding inside the brain can be insidious. A subdural hematoma can take hours to months to become evident.

There are three bleeding conditions inside the skull: epidural hematoma, subdural hematoma, and subarachnoid bleeding. Each condition is serious and life threatening. But, how can the prehospital care provider differentiate between the three? The prehospital care provider can help identify the nature of the problem based on their respective signs and symptoms. The following table highlights the differences among the three conditions based on their signs and symptoms.

Signs and Symptoms of Intracranial Bleeding Conditions

Epidural Hematoma	Subdural Hematoma	Subarachnoid Bleed
Arterial bleeding	Venous bleeding	Arterial bleeding
Above dura mater	Below dura mater	Deep inside brain
Recent head injury	Past head injury	No head injury
Rapid onset	Days to weeks in onset	Rapid onset
Skull fracture present	No skull fracture	No skull fracture
Initial loss of consciousness	No initial loss of consciousness	No initial loss of consciousness
Lucid interval then deterioration	Gradual deterioration	Rapid deterioration
Headache	Headache	Sudden, severe, headache

When the prehospital care provider encounters a patient with ominous complaints of a worsening headache, delirium, elevated blood pressure, and other findings associated with head injury, the provider should ask about a recent fall or blow to the head. If the medical history indicates a recent fall or head injury, the prehospital care provider should suspect intracranial bleeding.

Treatment for the subdural hematoma includes high-flow oxygen, elevation of the head, and prompt transportation to the emergency department. Spinal precautions may be necessary depending on the recency and mechanism of injury.

DECUBITUS ULCERS (BEDSORES)

After a fall or debilitating injury, the patient may become immobile. Due to changes in the circulation of the skin and reduction of collagen support for the blood vessels, immobility can lead to the development of decubitus ulcers, or bedsores. At some time, the prehospital care provider will be called on to care for and transport a patient with bedsores.

Decubitus ulcers are caused by pressure on the skin over a bony area. With aging, circulation to the skin decreases. Pressure on the skin near a bony prominence further reduces blood flow to the tissues. This can cause the skin to break down, allowing an ulcer to form. In tissue exposed to high pressures, a bedsore can begin in only 2 hours.

For most people, the pressure on the skin will eventually cause discomfort. The person will change position to reduce pressure on the area, restoring circulation. In the immobile or debilitated patient, the pressure is not relieved and an ulcer develops. Skin breakdown can occur more quickly in those patients with bladder or bowel incontinence. Typical areas for bedsores to develop include the buttocks, especially at the area of the sacrum and coccyx, and the hips, heels, ankles, and elbows.

Also consider the shearing forces placed on a patient's skin when the head of the bed or gurney is elevated. The weight of the body slides the patient down, placing significant shearing forces on the tailbone area (i.e., coccyx and sacrum). These shearing forces may contribute to the formation of bedsores.

There are four stages of decubitus ulcers based on the characteristics of the injury. Stage I consists of irritation of the skin. It is warm to the touch and appears red and unbroken. The skin does not blanch or turn pale with gentle finger pressure. Stage II involves a superficial breakdown of the skin surface. The upper layers of the skin, the epidermis and dermis, begin to deteriorate. The appearance is similar to an abrasion, blister, or shallow crater. Stage III ulcers are deeper. They include the subcutaneous fat and may expose the underlying muscle. A Stage III ulcer appears as a large crater. Stage IV sores are the worst, with damage extending through the skin down to the bone, muscle, joint, and tendons in the area. The following list summarizes the characteristics of each stage.

Stage I   Warm, red, unbroken skin. Skin does not blanch to the touch.

Stage II   Superficial deterioration of the epidermis and/or dermis. Appears as an abrasion, blister, or small crater.

Stage III Involves the skin and subcutaneous fat, exposing the muscle. Appears as a deep crater.

Stage IV   Extensive destruction of the skin and includes damage to the bone, muscle, joints, and tendons.

The ulcer can be a source of bacterial contamination. Bacteria, including staphylococcus, may be present in the wound. Use universal precautions when handling the patient with bedsores. The prehospital care provider will not be called to the scene because of the pressure ulcers. However, the prehospital care provider may encounter them while providing care for another condition. The prehospital care provider can provide some care for the ulcers by relieving the pressure on the site. Placing the patient on their side alleviates pressure from the coccyx. Elevating the patient's heels by placing padding under the calves of the patient's legs eliminates pressure on the feet and heels. If time and the patient's condition permit, apply a moist dressing to the ulcer prior to transporting the patient.

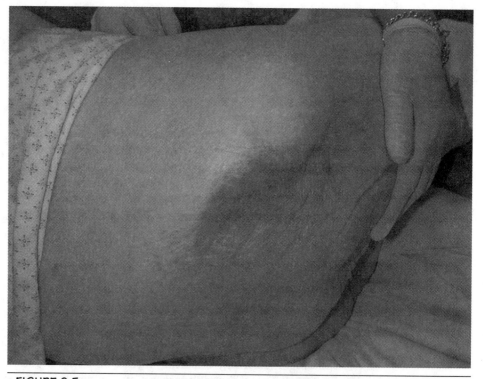

• FIGURE 9-5

Stage I decubitus ulcer is characterized by redness over the site. The skin is intact.
Source: Courtesy of Charles Stewart, MD FACEP; www.storysmith.net.

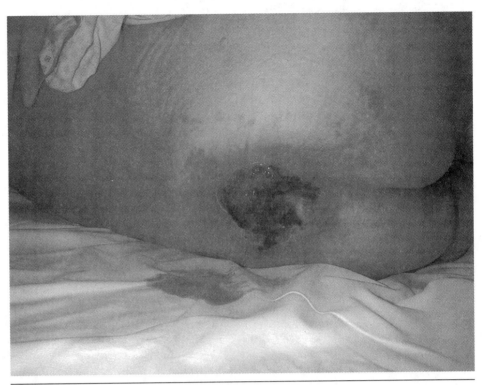

• FIGURE 9-6
Stage IV decubitus ulcer is characterized by tissue destruction involving muscle and perhaps bone.
Source: Courtesy of Charles Stewart, MD FACEP; www.storysmith.net.

KEY POINT

Decubitus ulcers can develop quickly and may be extremely difficult to heal.

BURNS

Decreased mobility can also result in other accidents. A very serious problem in the elderly patient is a burn injury. Because of the changes associated with aging, burns can cause more tissue destruction in the older adult. The elderly person may sustain a burn injury while cooking. Due to instability in gait, the senior may spill hot food or water onto their body or clothing. The risk of fire is also increased. Loose clothing around a hot stove or falling asleep while smoking has resulted in a number of critical burns to older adults. One source of burns that is often overlooked is hot water from the tap. If the water heater thermostat is set too high, water from a kitchen or bathroom faucet can scald the unsuspecting person. Thermal burns in the elderly can also be caused by falling asleep while using a heating pad or by sitting too close to a heating device such as a portable heater.

Older patients have a higher incidence of morbidity and mortality from burns than younger adults, probably due to overall health of younger adults and their ability to recover from an intense insult to the body. After suffering from a burn involving 30 percent of total body surface area, the survival rates of different age groups are startlingly different. People aged 5 to 34 years of age had a greater than 90 percent chance of survival. Those between the ages of 60 and 74 years had just over a 40 percent chance of survival. People over the age of 75 years had around a 10 percent survival rate. Thus, older patients are considered high risk. High-risk patients also include those with other medical conditions such as heart, liver, and kidney diseases. As can be seen by the table below, older adults can fit into several of the categories that place them at high risk for morbidity and mortality from burn injuries.

High-Risk Groups for Burn Injuries

Young children (< 2 years of age)
Older adults (> 65 years of age)
History of pulmonary disease
History of kidney disease
History of liver disease
History of metabolic disease
People with other major injuries

KEY POINT

The elderly and the frail are at a high risk for burns.

Burns are classified based on the degree of burn and the total body surface area involved. Since minor burns are discussed in EMS textbooks and do not pose a serious problem for the older adult, this section will only cover severe and critical burns. Similarly, this section will not discuss the visual appearance of first-, second-, and third-degree burns, since that information is also covered in detail in EMS reference textbooks.

Severe burns consist of third-degree burns covering more than 10 percent of total body surface area (TBSA) or second-degree burns that cover more than 15 percent TBSA. Second-degree burns of the face, hands, feet, and genitals are also considered severe burns.

Critical burns consist of second-degree burns covering more than 30 percent TBSA or third-degree burns covering more than 5 percent TBSA. Airway or inhalation burns are also considered critical burns. The classification guidelines for severe and critical burns are presented in the following table.

Classification of Severe and Critical Burns

Severe Burns	Critical Burns
Third-degree burns > 10% TBSA	Second-degree burns > 30% TBSA
Second-degree burns > 15% TBSA	Third-degree burns > 5% TBSA
Burns on hands, feet, face, perineum	Inhalation burns

After stopping the burning process by removing the source of heat or by dousing any burning clothing, prehospital care of the burn patient initially includes assessing and maintaining a patent airway. Always consider and look for an airway burn in a victim with thermal burns. Administer high-flow oxygen and consider advanced airway support such as endotracheal intubation. Intubation of the burn patient should be seriously considered when the patient has sustained full-thickness burns to the lips or a full-thickness burn that goes around the neck. If the patient has burns on the palate or tongue, intubation may be needed for airway management.

Assess the severity of the burn and try to determine the total body surface area involved. Using the "Rule of 9s" is a reasonably easy way to assess the extent of injury (see the following figure). The TBSA along with the patient's weight can be used to determine fluid resuscitation.

Fluid resuscitation may begin in the prehospital setting. There are a few different formulas for determining the amount of fluid to be administered over the first 8 to 24 hours after the burn injury. A simple and easy-to-use formula is the Parkland formula. The calculations are simple, and fluid resuscitation can be initiated in the field. The Parkland formula is based upon the percent TBSA and the patient's weight. Using a crystalloid solution such as lactated Ringer's solution, initiate large-bore IV therapy and administer the solution as follows:

$$4 \text{ ml lactated Ringer's} \times \%\text{TBSA} \times \text{weight (kg)}$$

For example, a 150-pound (68-kg patient) with 25 percent TBSA should receive:

$$4 \text{ ml} \times 25 \times 68 = 6,800 \text{ ml of fluid over the first 24 hours.}$$

The solution is given in divided amounts, with the first half given during the first 8 hours and the remainder administered over the next 16 hours. The total quantity looks large, and at first glance it seems that the IV solution administration set would be set to fully open. This is not the case. Using the preceding example, the patient would receive 425 mls of solution over the first hour after the injury. That equates to a fraction over 7 mls per minute. Using a standard solution administration set (10 drops/ml), the prehospital care provider would infuse 70 drops of IV solution per minute. This rate is just over one drop per second and is easy to titrate.

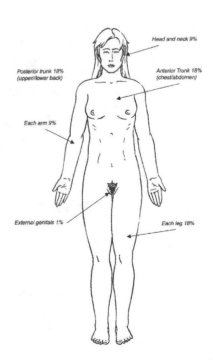

• FIGURE 9-7

Rule of nines in burn assessment.

Source: Courtesy Brady *MedEMT,* p. 137.

Complications associated with fluid resuscitation include overhydrating the patient, especially in the patient with underlying cardiac or renal disease. Monitor the patient for fluid overload and lower the rate of infusion should the patient show signs of fluid overload. More than likely, in the prehospital setting and limited time with the patient, signs of fluid overload will not be seen.

Be aware of the complications associated with burns and provide additional therapy as needed. For example, the burn patient may become hypothermic due to their inability to regulate body temperature or because of additional heat loss due to the evaporation of body fluids from burned areas. Maintain body heat with sheets or blankets to minimize heat loss.

CARBON MONOXIDE POISONING

Carbon monoxide poisoning is another potential hazard for older adults. Faulty gas or oil furnaces, portable kerosene-burning heaters, and fireplaces can cause carbon monoxide poisoning. Additional sources of carbon monoxide poisoning are more subtle. For example, an elderly couple on a fixed income worries about the high cost of heating their home. So, rather than using the furnace, they bring the portable hibachi grill inside and burn charcoal to heat the room. Without proper ventilation, carbon monoxide can accumulate, with serious consequences. Another example is even more insidious. Prior to leaving the home on a cold winter's day, an older couple starts their car inside the garage. Even though the garage door is partially open, the couple succumbs to carbon monoxide poisoning. The source of the carbon monoxide was later identified as the furnace that was located inside the garage. While the car was running, the car exhaust was being drawn into the house through the furnace.

Since carbon monoxide poisoning can be obvious or hidden, the prehospital care provider should be alert to its possibility. During the winter months, a sudden onset of severe headache, nausea, vomiting, and confusion should trigger questions about indoor heaters or exposure to vehicle exhaust. Patients may also complain of difficulty breathing since carbon monoxide has a 200 to 250 times greater affinity for hemoglobin than oxygen. In high levels, the poison interferes with the release of oxygen to the tissues. While considered classic, the cherry-red skin color of those suffering from carbon monoxide exposure is a late finding, and usually occurs when the carbon monoxide levels are high and death is near or has already occurred. Cyanosis is more typical in the earlier stages of carbon monoxide poisoning.

Signs and Symptoms of Carbon Monoxide Poisoning

Severe headache

Nausea

Vomiting

Confusion or delirium

Dyspnea

Cyanosis

Cherry-red skin color (late finding)

Coma

Death

Treatment for carbon monoxide poisoning includes immediate evacuation from the area and administration of high-flow oxygen. If necessary and available, intubation may be required to support ventilation. Transportation to the emergency department should not be delayed.

SUMMARY

Falls and injuries occur easily in the older patient due to a number of factors including faltering gait, altered mentation, osteoporosis, and other things. The senior's quality of life after a fall is severely affected and, after a hip fracture, it can quickly deteriorate. Annually, the cost of caring for older victims of fall injuries approaches $70 billion.

This chapter has addressed accidental injuries in the older adult including falls, hip fractures, decubitus ulcers, burns, and carbon monoxide poisoning. It has also addressed some of the mechanisms of injury in the senior citizen. By understanding the nature and potential risk of these injuries as well as properly caring for the patient, the prehospital care provider can reduce the morbidity and mortality of accidental injuries in the senior citizen.

ON THE JOB

You are called to a shopping mall in the middle of the afternoon to attend to a 69-year-old woman who, bystanders state, suddenly fell. You approach the woman who appears embarrassed by all the attention she is receiving from mall security and passers-by. The woman tells you that she suddenly became dizzy and collapsed. She doesn't remember exactly what happened since "things happened so fast." The woman tells you that, after she fell, she felt fine while sitting on the floor. Physical assessment reveals soft tissue injury to her right hip with no indication of fracture. The woman's vital signs are BP–110/70, P–68, R–18 and nonlabored. She tells you that her blood pressure seems low, but her doctor had put her on labetalol to lower her blood pressure from 180/110. Discuss reasons for the woman's fall. What contributed to her dizziness? If the woman had sustained a fractured hip, how would you treat the injury?

10

Fall and Injury Prevention

OBJECTIVES

At the end of the chapter, the reader will be able to:

1. List eight risk factors for falling.
2. Other than a home safety evaluation, list three things that can decrease an older adult's risk of falling.
3. Describe two hazards outside of the home that increase the risk for falling.
4. List six hazards inside the home that increase the risk for falling.
5. Describe how an older adult can compensate for hard-to-reach items located in a kitchen cupboard.
6. Describe how improperly fitting clothes can contribute to a fall.
7. List three things that can prevent fires, burns, and scald injuries.

Falls and injuries related to falls account for numerous deaths in the United States annually. Older adults are more likely to sustain a fall and fall-related injury than are younger adults. Although all falls do not result in injury or hospitalization, they can lead to a fear of falling which, in turn, leads to a decrease in activity which, in turn, leads to a drop in self-confidence which, in turn, heightens the fear of falling! This can become a vicious cycle. Since EMS is a community service, implementation of a fall and injury prevention program for the area's older population would benefit both seniors as well as the EMS agency. The following information can be used in a fall and injury prevention program.

KEY POINT

EMS agencies should provide fall and injury prevention programs to the elderly citizens of the community.

In addition to the causes of falls discussed in Chapter 9, risk factors for falling include:

- Use of sedative-type medications
- History of a previous fall, especially if the prior fall was recent
- Impaired cognition
- Visual impairment
- Disability involving one or both legs
- Gait problems
- Pain or other problem in one or both feet
- Safety hazards in the home

PREVENTING FALLS AND INJURIES

Before discussing home safety hazards and suggestions for correcting them, consider other factors that can reduce the risk of injury. These other factors include exercise, review of prescription and nonprescription medications, and a vision examination.

Exercise

Getting some exercise is one of the more important things a senior can do to reduce the risk of falling. Exercise builds and maintains muscle tone. Additionally, exercise increases a person's stamina and makes the person generally feel better. Exercise also improves a person's self-confidence in their ability to avoid falling. Without exercise, muscles weaken and the chance of falling increases.

Review All Medications

With the help of the doctor or pharmacist, all medications—prescription and nonprescription—should be reviewed. Medications that cause drowsiness, weakness, fatigue, or confusion should be avoided, if possible. Watch for drug interactions. Some medications used in combination with others can increase the risk of falls or injuries.

Have a Complete Vision Examination

Have the eyes checked for visual acuity, including refraction, glaucoma, cataracts, macular degeneration, and other eye diseases. Treat problems if possible, and, if vision is impaired, conduct a thorough home safety evaluation.

Once an exercise regimen has been established, the medications reviewed, and the eyes checked, the older adult should assess the home for safety hazards. There are a number of checklists available to help in this process. A checklist from CDC has been included in the Appendix for reference and use.

There are a number of safety hazards in the home that can be easily discovered and corrected. When checking for safety hazards, assess the outside of the residence as well as the inside.

Safety Hazard Checklist

Hazard	**Corrective Action**
Clutter on the walkways or sidewalks	Remove clutter and keep the area clean
Clearly marked steps or irregular walkways	Use paint or reflective tape to mark steps or irregular walkways

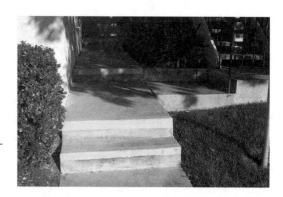

• FIGURE 10-1
Examine safety of steps.

Loose steps or railings (including inside stairways)	Secure railings, steps, and banisters as needed

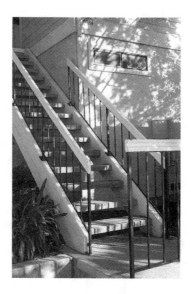

• FIGURE 10-2
Examine stairs and railing for safety.

Hazard	Corrective Action
Lighting around doorways and stairwells	Repair broken fixtures, replace burned out lights, and add new lights to ensure safety
Entry door facing	Use paint or reflective tape to highlight
	Use plywood to make a ramp if needed
Loose rugs on floors	Use double-stick tape to attach rugs to floor

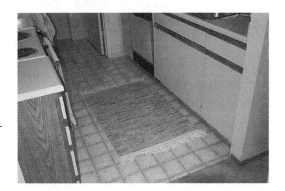

• FIGURE 10-3
Use double-stick carpet tape to secure a loose rug to the floor.

Hazard	Corrective Action
Water or oils on floor	Mop and clean spills as soon as possible
Poor lighting	Replace broken fixtures, replace burned out lights, add nightlights in bedrooms and bathrooms
Bed so high that it might cause the senior to fall when getting out of bed	Replace or remove the bed frame to lower the bed closer to floor
Overstuffed chairs difficult to exit	Replace overstuffed chairs or get an elevator lift to help the senior get out of the chair
Chairs with wheels	Remove wheels or replace wheeled chairs
Tripping over loose clothes	Make sure clothing properly fits. Use nonslip pads on soles of shoes
Tripping over exposed extension cord	Cover cord with rug or route around walls

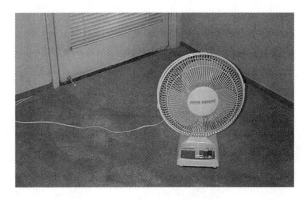

• FIGURE 10-4
Cover exposed extension cords.

Hazard

Slippery bathtubs

Corrective Action

Install railings and a skid-proof mat

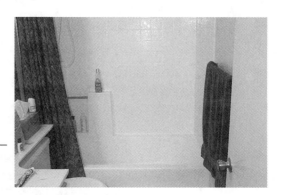

• FIGURE 10-5
Install safety rails and non-slip mat.

Hazard

Difficulty getting off the toilet

Items in cupboards are hard to reach

Corrective Action

Use a 3:1 commode over the toilet to permit easier standing from the toilet stool

Move items to a lower shelf or purchase a "grabbing" device. Use caution with step stool

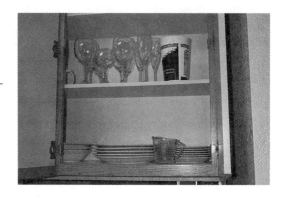

• FIGURE 10-6
Items in cabinet should be within easy reach. A small step stool can be used to help reach more difficult items. Step stools should be very sturdy.

Poor vision

Wear appropriate glasses and hold handrail when climbing stairs. Do not carry too many items at one time

Impaired hearing prevents alarms such as smoke and fire alarms from being heard

Make sure audible warnings such as smoke and fire alarms have lights that turn on when the alarm sounds

Inappropriate use of walking aids such as canes and walkers

Seek professional training from physical therapist on use of device. Make sure devices are properly fitted. Get help when walking.

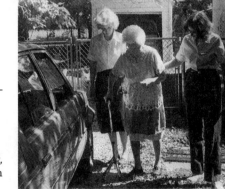

• FIGURE 10-7

Use appropriate walking aids and get help when ambulating.

Source: Photo courtesy on *Aging,* a magazine of the Administration on Aging.

In addition to exercising, reviewing medications, and getting a comprehensive vision examination, there are some general safety tips for seniors. These tips include information on clothing, being alert to changes in the weather, and fire, burn, and scald prevention.

Suitable Clothing

Make sure clothing fits properly and cannot fall off and cause tripping

Pants should be a suitable length

Do not wear slippers or sandals outside of the home

Apply nonslip pads to soles of shoes or use rubber-soled shoes

Be Aware of Potential Changes in the Weather

Get a weather report every day

Keep the house cool and well ventilated during warm months. Keep adequately hydrated by drinking eight cups of water daily

Avoid prolonged exposure to heat and the sun

Keep warm in cooler months by eating right, consuming hot food with high calories

Keep the house warm in cooler months and use sweaters to ensure warmth

Portable heaters should be used with caution

Exercise indoors on particularly warm or cold days

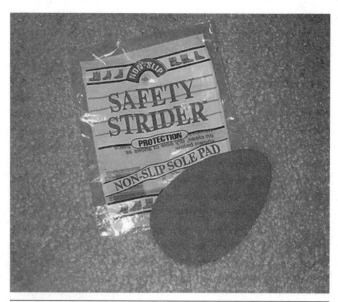

• FIGURE 10-8

Abrasive pads that adhere to the soles of the shoes will increase traction and reduce falls.

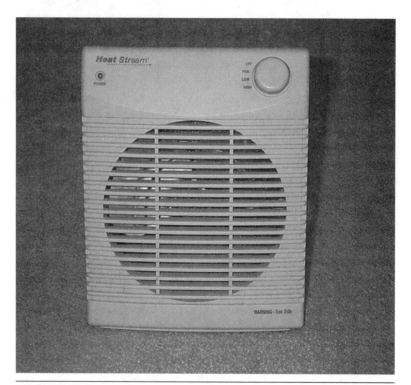

• FIGURE 10-9

Portable heaters should be kept a safe distance from furniture, drapes, and frail skin. They should also have an automatic shutoff in the event the heater tips over.

Prevent Fires, Burns, and Scald Injuries

Prevent stove-top spills, especially those involving oils or combustible materials

Keep a fire extinguisher in the kitchen

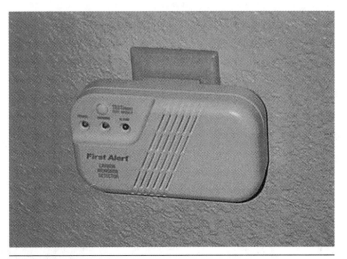

• FIGURE 10-10
Along with smoke detectors, be sure to install a carbon monoxide detector.

Use a portable heater with an automatic shutoff in case it tips over

Make sure that portable kerosene heaters are checked for carbon monoxide

Install a carbon monoxide detector

Carry hot items using gloves or a towel

Use a whistling-type teapot when boiling water

Keep the water heater thermostat no higher than 120°F.

SUMMARY

This chapter has focused on fall and injury prevention tips that will enable the prehospital care provider to provide safety and fall prevention training within the community or to inspect the home of a senior citizen to identify and eliminate safety hazards.

ON THE JOB

You are called to a retirement condominium community where you are greeted by an elderly woman who told you her husband fell. The woman escorts you up a flight of stairs to the apartment. As she climbs the stairs, the woman tends to lean against the wall of the building for support because there is no railing to hold. Once inside the apartment, you find her husband, a 78-year-old man, lying supine on the living room floor. As you approach the man, you note the kitchen is a mess with dirty dishes piled in the sink, a throw rug crumpled on the floor, and a overflowing trash can. Around the living room, you see old newspapers piled in one corner. A fan, connected to an extension cord, cools an overly warm room; a portable heater is also connected to the same extension cord. Because you are aware that home safety is important for the older adult, list the unsafe things identified while viewing the entire scene. After caring for the man's injuries, what can you advise the couple to do to make their home safe?

11

End-Stage Renal Disease

OBJECTIVES

At the end of the chapter, the reader will be able to:

1 Define chronic renal failure.
2 Define end-stage renal disease.
3 List 10 signs or symptoms of chronic renal disease.
4 List 12 signs or symptoms of end-stage renal disease.
5 Describe the three access routes used to perform hemodialysis.
6 Describe how peritoneal dialysis differs from hemodialysis.
7 List three steps taken to minimize clotting of the access route.
8 Describe the procedure for controlling external bleeding from a disconnected shunt.
9 List four signs of fluid overload in the dialysis patient.
10 Describe the appearance of the ECG in a patient with hyperkalemia.

Dialysate   Fluid used in peritoneal dialysis to remove excess fluids, wastes, and toxins from the blood.

Dialyzer   The machine or membrane used in the dialysis machine to remove excess fluids, wastes, and toxins from the blood during hemodialysis.

Electrolytes   A chemical that, when dissolved in water, forms ions and is able to conduct electricity or electric current. Some of the body's electrolytes include sodium, potassium, and calcium.

Fistula   A surgically created passage between an artery and a vein for the purpose of hemodialysis treatment.

Graft   In hemodialysis, a blood vessel from the patient or a cow or a synthetic device used to connect an artery and vein to allow access for hemodialysis.

Hemodialysis   Procedure in which the patient's blood is removed and filtered of excess fluids, waste, and toxins, and then returned to the patient.

Hemostats   A type of clamp used to seal blood vessels or plastic tubing. The name means "to stop bleeding."

Hyperkalemia   An excessive amount of potassium in the patient's body.

Lethargy   A state of feeling sluggish or indifferent. It can also mean stupor or coma.

Peripheral edema   Tissue swelling in the extremities due to excess fluid seeping from the blood vessels into the tissues.

Pulmonary edema   Fluid in the alveoli caused by excessive fluid or the heart's inability to effectively pump blood from the body to the heart.

Peritoneal dialysis   A procedure that uses the lining of the abdominal cavity (peritoneum) to filter fluids, waste, and toxins from the blood.

Shunt   In hemodialysis, the use of catheters to connect an artery and vein. The catheters are inserted through the skin and used to remove and return blood that is being filtered. The catheters are connected to each other when not in use for hemodialysis.

Uremic frost   Condition where dried crystals of urea are found on the skin, giving the patient a frosted appearance.

CHRONIC RENAL FAILURE AND END-STAGE RENAL DISEASE

A large number of older adults develop what is known as end-stage renal disease (ESRD). The disease occurs when the kidneys fail to excrete waste, concentrate urine, and regulate the body's electrolytes. Initially, the patient develops chronic renal failure, which is when the kidneys have lost 60 percent of their ability to function. As the kidneys continue to fail over time, the patient develops ESRD. The treatments for ESRD are dialysis or kidney transplantation. Without dialysis or kidney transplantation, the patient's life is in jeopardy. It is important to be aware of ESRD, since prehospital care providers will be called to care for and transport patients with this condition or those who have complications of ESRD and its treatment. The reason for the call to 9-1-1 may be associated with ESRD or it may be for a totally separate reason. The purpose of this chapter is to discuss chronic renal failure and ESRD, as well as hemodialysis and peritoneal dialysis. The chapter will also discuss complications associated with dialysis.

It is estimated that four out of 10,000 people in the United States have ESRD, and that 100,000 are currently receiving treatment by dialysis. Many of these patients have a long history of diabetes, however, there are other causes of ESRD. Conditions such as untreated hypertension, inflammation of the kidneys (glomerulonephritis), and long-term exposure to analgesics have been known to permanently damage the kidneys.

KEY POINT

Diabetes, hypertension, and glomerulonephritis are a few of the causes of end-stage renal disease (ESRD).

Since chronic renal failure is slow in onset, the signs and symptoms may not immediately bring to mind kidney failure. The signs and symptoms of chronic renal failure are presented in the following list.

Signs and Symptoms of Chronic Renal Failure

Headache

Weakness

Lethargy

Loss of appetite

Vomiting

Increased urination (the kidneys cannot conserve water)

Rusty- or brown-colored urine

Increased thirst (loss of water leads to dehydration)

Hypertension

Puffiness around the eyes

Patients with chronic renal failure who are under medical supervision have frequent physical examinations, blood pressure evaluations, and blood tests and receive medications for hypertension.

When the patient develops ESRD, additional signs and symptoms may appear. These signs and symptoms are mild until kidney function is 15 percent or less of normal and include:

Confusion

Decreased levels of consciousness

Dyspnea

Peripheral edema

Chest pain

Bone pain

Itching skin

Nausea and vomiting

Diarrhea

Easy bruising

Muscle twitching

Seizures

DIALYSIS

Patients with ESRD receive dialysis treatments until a transplant can be arranged. For the older adult, a transplant may not be a viable option due to advancing age, concurrent medical conditions, or cost. Thus, the patient is on life-long dialysis.

> **KEY POINT**
>
> Patients with ESRD must undergo dialysis until and if a kidney transplant can be performed.

There are two types of dialysis treatments available—hemodialysis and peritoneal dialysis. Hemodialysis is usually performed at a clinic, but some home machines are available. Peritoneal dialysis is performed in the home.

HEMODIALYSIS

Hemodialysis is a procedure that cleans and filters the blood by removing waste products and fluids. To accomplish this, the blood is filtered through a machine called a dialyzer. Once the blood is filtered, it is returned to the patient. The

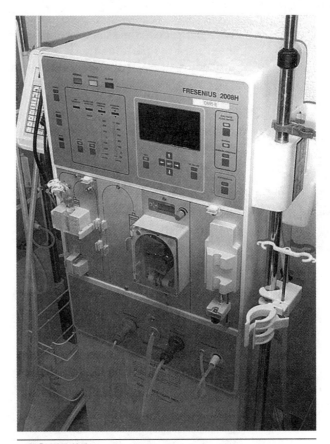

• FIGURE 11-1
Hemodialysis machines such as this filter wastes and toxins from the blood of a patient with ESRD.

patient's blood is accessed by shunt, graft, or fistula. With a shunt, which is typically used while waiting for other access routes to heal, catheters are inserted into an artery and a vein from outside the body. Most shunts are located on the forearm. When not in use to dialyze a patient, the catheters are connected to each other with clear tubing, allowing the continuous flow of blood from artery to vein. The catheters are then covered with self-adhering roller gauze for protection. Implementation of the two other access routes requires surgery. For a graft, a surgeon will connect a piece of the patient's saphenous vein (from the patient's leg) to an artery and vein. In lieu of using the patient's own blood vessel, a cow's artery or a synthetic graft can be used. In creating a fistula, an artery and vein in the arm or leg are surgically connected to each other under the skin. After healing, the graft or the fistula can be used to withdraw blood from and return it to the patient. Hemodialysis is generally performed three times per week and takes from 2 to 5 hours per treatment.

> ### KEY POINT
>
> Patients on hemodialysis will have a shunt, graft, or fistula connecting an artery and vein. The shunt, graft, or fistula, provides access to the patient's blood so that it can be removed, filtered, and returned.

PERITONEAL DIALYSIS

With peritoneal dialysis, the dialysis procedure is performed at home. The treatment uses the peritoneum in the abdomen to filter and cleanse the blood. The procedure uses a catheter that has been surgically implanted into the abdomen.

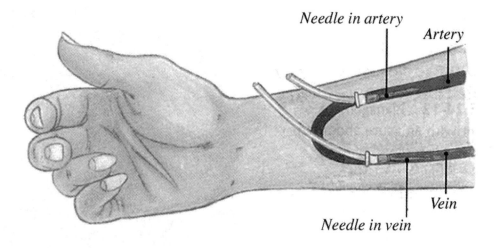

Needle in artery

Artery

Vein

Needle in vein

• FIGURE 11-2
A shunt is a plastic tube that connects an artery and vein.
Source: Courtesy Brady *Emergency Care,* p. 788.

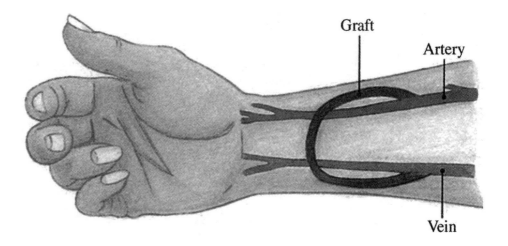

Graft

Artery

Vein

• FIGURE 11-3
A graft connects an artery to a vein.
Source: Courtesy Brady *Emergency Care,* p. 788.

Once the catheter is ready to use, it is attached to a bag of solution called dialysate that is infused into the abdomen.

In one form of peritoneal dialysis called continuous ambulatory peritoneal dialysis, after the solution has been administered, the catheter is sealed and covered, and the patient retains the dialysate in the abdomen for several hours. After a specified time, usually 4 to 6 hours, the dialysate, which has cleansed and filtered the blood, is drained. This method of peritoneal dialysis is performed daily and repeated four to five times per day.

Another form of peritoneal dialysis performed at home is called continuous cycle peritoneal dialysis. The procedure is essentially the same as the procedure described for continuous ambulatory peritoneal dialysis, however, with this method, the patient's catheter connects to a machine that automatically fills and drains the dialysate. This procedure is generally done at night and takes from 10 to 12 hours to complete.

KEY POINT

Peritoneal dialysis uses a catheter inserted into the abdomen to filter waste products from the blood.

PATIENT CARE

There are a few things prehospital care providers should remember when caring for a patient who receives dialysis treatments. These tips apply regardless of whether the call for assistance is related to the dialysis or if it is for some other

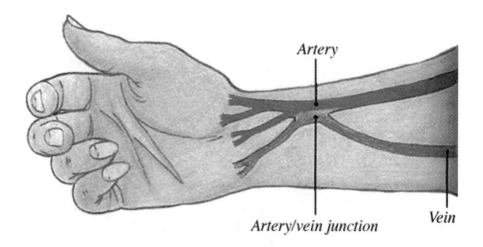

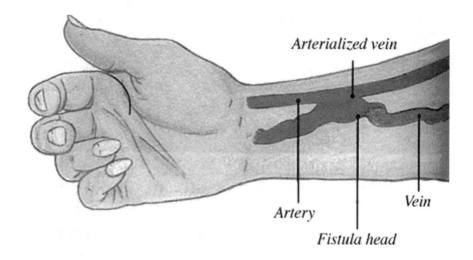

• FIGURE 11-4
A fistula is formed by surgically connecting an artery to a vein.
Source: Courtesy Brady *Emergency Care,* p. 788.

medical emergency. Following these guidelines will prevent inadvertent clotting of the graft or fistula.

- Do not take the patient's blood pressure on the extremity with the access site. Some patients may have more than one graft or fistula because one of the access sites has failed. Ask which site is being used. If the patient is unable to answer or is uncertain, gently touch the access site. The presence of a "thrill" or vibration to the touch indicates a patent site.
- Do not apply firm, direct pressure on the arm with the site, even if there is bleeding. Gentle pressure will usually suffice.
- Loosen tight or restrictive clothing on the extremity of the access site.

As mentioned earlier, the dialysis patient will use a shunt prior to the implantation of an internal access site. The shunt could clot or become dislodged or disconnected. Examine the plastic catheter for the blood color. Dark blood inside the tubing could indicate clotting.

If the catheter becomes dislodged, severe bleeding inside the extremity at the site will occur. Direct pressure followed by rapid transportation to the emergency department is the only available emergency treatment for this condition.

If the tubing becomes disconnected, use hemostats to clamp the tubing to control the bleeding. After the tubing has been clamped, transport the patient to the emergency department. If necessary, provide basic life-support treatment for shock.

COMPLICATIONS OF DIALYSIS

Prehospital care providers may be called to assist a dialysis patient who is suffering from complications of the treatment. The adverse effects of dialysis include hypotension, muscle cramps, nausea, and vomiting. Typically, these complications occur at the dialysis center where medical treatment is provided by the center's staff. EMS may be called to transport the patient to the emergency department. If the patient becomes hypotensive after leaving the dialysis treatment center or while being treated at home, prehospital care providers can provide basic life-support treatment for shock, including administering oxygen and elevating the patient's legs. Initiating IV therapy is not indicated.

Occasionally, there may be some bleeding at the catheter insertion site after a dialysis treatment. Should this occur, apply gentle pressure to the area, cover it with a sterile dressing, and transport the patient to the emergency department.

For patients on peritoneal dialysis, infection at the catheter site could lead to peritonitis or sepsis. If peritonitis is suspected, immediate transportation to the emergency department is required.

Occasionally, a patient is unable to complete a dialysis treatment due to complications during therapy. These patients are returned home until the next treatment. Usually, the patients are advised to closely monitor their diet and fluid intake to avoid serious and potentially life-threatening health problems associated with fluid overload, waste accumulation, and electrolyte imbalance. Signs and symptoms of fluid overload include acute pulmonary edema, hypertensive crisis, an elevated blood potassium level (hyperkalemia), and uremic frost.

Pulmonary edema and hypertensive crisis caused by fluid overload in patients with ESRD are similar to pulmonary edema and hypertensive crisis from other conditions. With very high potassium levels, the patient may develop asystole without warning. Physical signs and symptoms of hyperkalemia include a slow, irregular pulse; muscular weakness; and tingling of the hands, feet, and tongue. The ECG of a patient with hyperkalemia will have a depressed P-wave, a widened QRS complex, and peaked T-waves.

Uremic frost is created when the body tries to rid excess urea through sweating. When the perspiration dries, it leaves a crystal residue on the skin that resembles a frost and smells like urine.

Signs and Symptoms of Fluid Overload

Pulmonary edema

Hypertension

Hyperkalemia

Uremic frost

When called to assist a patient in acute distress from fluid overload, the prehospital care provider is faced with a dilemma. Taking a blood pressure may be "iffy" depending on the location of the access site. Initiating an IV is not indicated since the patient has too much fluid volume. Administration of a diuretic is contraindicated since the patient's kidneys do not work. The most effective treatment is to monitor the airway and administer high-flow supplemental oxygen, prepare to intubate the patient and assist ventilation, and monitor the patient's ECG. Be prepared to initiate CPR in the event of asystole. Prior to transporting the patient, determine the location of the closest hospital with dialysis capabilities. Transporting the patient to a close emergency department that has no dialysis capabilities may waste precious time.

KEY POINT

Be aware of potential complications of dialysis such as bleeding from the access site, a disconnected shunt, fluid overload, and hyperkalemia.

SUMMARY

This chapter has highlighted a condition that can threaten the life of the older adult—end-stage renal disease. Without dialysis or kidney transplantation, the patient with ESRD will eventually die. Although prehospital care providers may not be called to care for these patients as often as those with other medical complaints, prehospital care providers need to be aware of the condition, its treatment, and the complications of the disease and its treatments. Since prehospital treatment options are severely limited, knowing the nature and effects of the disease can guide the prehospital care provider in their emergency care options.

Patients with ESRD must be dialyzed in order to survive. Failure to adequately remove excess water, wastes, and toxins can result in fluid overload with potentially life-threatening effects on the cardiovascular system. Prompt recognition of the condition along with rapid transportation to a facility with dialysis capabilities can save the patient's life.

ON THE JOB

At 7:10 A.M., you receive a call for difficult breathing. You arrive at a private residence where a distraught woman escorts you to the patient's room. You find a 68-year-old man lying supine on his bed. He is unresponsive to verbal or physical stimulation. The woman tells you her husband has been on dialysis for 2 years and had a treatment 2 days ago that he did not tolerate well. Because he became ill, they dialysis treatment ended early. The woman also tells you that she and her husband were at a barbecue yesterday where he consumed a lot of watermelon. You notice that the patient has pulmonary edema and that his skin has dried crystals that smell like urine. Describe how you would care for this patient. What are the effects of hyperkalemia on the heart? Could you give diuretics to treat the pulmonary edema?

12

The Terminally Ill Patient

OBJECTIVES

At the end of the chapter, the reader will be able to:

1 Discuss four purposes of hospice care.
2 List seven steps that can be taken to allow the patient to die with dignity.
3 Describe 11 things that happen as the body prepares to die.
4 Describe what is meant by a living will.
5 Describe what is meant by durable power of attorney for healthcare.
6 Define Do Not Resuscitate (DNR).
7 Explain that DNR does not mean withholding care and comfort.
8 List five general procedures when dealing with a DNR order in the prehospital setting.

WORDS TO KNOW

Do Not Resuscitate (DNR)   Withholding CPR, ventilation, defibrillation, and medication therapy in the event a patient develops cardiac or respiratory arrest.

Cheyne-Stokes breathing   A waxing and waning of breathing followed by periods of apnea.

Febrile   Having an elevated body temperature or fever.

Hospice   Facility or program that eases the final days of the terminally ill patient.

Hallucinations   A perception of something sensory that has no basis in reality or no basis in external stimulation. Hallucinations can involve any of the five senses.

Incontinence   Inability to control the bladder or bowel.

Lividity   Discoloration similar to a bruise caused by gravitation (settling) of blood.

INTRODUCTION

EMS personnel primarily respond to medical emergencies to provide acute care to the critically ill or injured patient. Prehospital care providers are also often called to provide care and transportation on a nonemergency basis. Some of these calls involve patients who are terminally ill and some that have been placed in hospice care. When some patients reach the end of life, they may wish to be transported to an in-patient hospice so that they do not die at home. Or, they may wish to be taken from an in-patient hospice or hospital to their home to be with family when the end arrives. Prehospital care providers are often called on to provide such services. It should also be noted that prehospital care providers might be home with a terminally ill relative when death arrives. The purpose of this chapter is to present an overview of hospice care, highlight the care of the dying patient, and discuss Do Not Resuscitate (DNR) orders, advanced directives, and durable powers of attorney (DPOA) as they apply to prehospital care.

HOSPICE

By definition, hospice means a program that eases the last days of the terminally ill patient. Some hospice programs consist of in-patient facilities, whereas other programs provide care for the dying patient at home. Perhaps it would be best to consider hospice care as a mindset as opposed to a location or program. Patients are placed into hospice care when the diagnosis and prognosis are clearly known. Typically, when there is no available cure and the patient's condition has or will deteriorate, a patient will enter a hospice program. When the patient enters the hospice, the patient's physician estimates that they have less than 6 months to live.

Hospice care serves several purposes, including:

- Offering care and support to the patient and family before, during, and after death.
- Providing relief of symptoms such as pain, nausea, dyspnea, and others to ensure the patient's comfort.
- Providing psychological support for the patient and family.
- Giving nutrition and hydration as appropriate and desired by the patient.

There is great fear in the patient that, by entering a hospice program, all support for pain relief, difficulty breathing, and medications will be stopped; that they will suffer as their life ends. This is not true. Pain relief, administration of medications, and relief from respiratory distress are all important components of the hospice program. Ultimately, the patient is in control of their care. Hospice patients have DNR orders and Advanced Directives in place, along with a signed DPOA for healthcare in the event the patient becomes too ill to verbally express their desires. DNR, advanced directives, and DPOA are discussed later in this chapter.

CARING FOR THE TERMINALLY ILL

When called to assist the terminally ill patient, there are several guidelines that will make contact with the dying patient easier on both the patient and the prehospital care provider. These guidelines are in addition to providing relief from pain and suffering.

- Be respectful of the patient and family. Show your respect by making eye contact with the patient and family.
- Touch the patient. The patient is dying and touch is reassuring. The dying patient is not contagious or infectious. When their hand is held or a hand is placed on their shoulder, the prehospital care provider is at minimal risk for contracting an infectious disease. Occasionally, the patient's condition or the treatment they received could be disfiguring. The patient may be emaciated and feel that their appearance is disgusting. Laying on of hands reassures and comforts the patient.
- Listen to the patient. Let the patient vent as needed. Show that you are listening and use empathic or active listening. Understand that the patient's emotional outbursts, while seemingly directed at you, should not be taken personally.
- If the patient or family has a particular religious belief, allow them to express it even if you do not share it. However, the prehospital care provider should not impose their own religious beliefs on the patient or the patient's family.
- Use the "Golden Rule." Ask, "If I were dying, what would I want from the prehospital care provider while being transported to or from a facility?"
- Learn about the grief process. Elisabeth Kubler-Ross broke important ground on dealing with death and dying. She identified the five stages of grief—denial, anger, bargaining, depression, and acceptance.
- Identify your own inner feelings and personal emotions about death and dying.

STAGES OF DYING

What happens when a patient dies? EMS personnel see patients die from sudden or acute conditions, but do not frequently see or provide care for the patient who is dying from a chronic illness. As the body begins to die, it prepares for the death sometimes several hours to several days before death occurs. The following changes that occur in the dying process are not listed in any particular order, and not all of these changes will occur. As in life, each person is unique in death.

As death approaches:

- The arms and legs become cool to the touch. Circulation slows and lividity can develop.
- Body temperature fluctuates from cool to normal to elevated. If the patient is febrile, aspirin or acetaminophen along with cool compresses can alleviate the fever.
- Sleep is increased and the patient may be difficult to arouse.
- When awake, the patient may be confused or disoriented. They may not recognize surroundings or family members.
- Hallucinations can develop. The dying patient may state that they have seen or spoken with deceased family members. The patient may actually be heard having a conversation with a deceased family member.
- Bowel and bladder incontinence occurs. Eventually, the kidneys shut down and the patient stops urinating.
- Appetite and thirst are diminished or absent.
- Saliva and secretions can pool in the mouth and throat. These secretions can cause noisy breathing. Suction the airway and mouth as needed.
- Hearing, vision, and speech are decreased. Speech may be unintelligible or incoherent. Remember that hearing is the last sense to be lost. Keep conversations around the patient appropriate. Do not assume that the comatose patient cannot hear you.
- Irregular breathing such as Cheyne-Stokes ventilation may develop. The patient is unaware of the change in breathing and the prehospital care provider need not do anything for the patient to correct the abnormal breathing.
- The patient lapses into a coma and death follows. However, some patients remain conscious until death.

KEY POINT

The comatose patient who is nearing death may still hear everything that is said. Keep conversations appropriate.

EMS RESPONSE IN DEATH AND DYING

Once death has occurred, EMS is no longer needed. In some areas, the local ambulance service may be used to transport the body to a local hospital for "pronouncement." Follow local protocols for the transportation of a patient's remains.

Occasionally, family members or staff at a skilled nursing facility will call 9-1-1 when the patient expires or when they are extremely close to death. This may be due to their not knowing the best procedures for handling the death. The family may have been instructed to call the police department when the patient dies. When calling 9-1-1 for police assistance, they may also activate an EMS response. In some cases, skilled nursing facility staff may feel that the patient should be in a hospital when dying. So, they call 9-1-1 to have the dying patient transported.

When responding to the report of a death or dying patient, prehospital care providers are faced with several challenges. The first challenge is to identify a situation in which a terminally ill patient has expired. A second challenge is to determine if a deceased person or dying patient has a DNR order or Advanced Directive regarding care.

ADVANCED DIRECTIVE AND DPOA

In 1991, Congress enacted the Patient Self-Determination Act that required healthcare facilities to inform patients of their rights to make decisions about their care. This is especially important if the patient becomes too ill to make informed decisions about care. With an advanced directive in place, a person has indicated what therapy they will accept and what treatment options they will refuse. Simply stated, each patient has the right to self-determination.

Advanced directives are also known as living wills, and provide information to healthcare workers on what therapy is acceptable and what therapy should not be performed. Advanced directives are generally put into place when the diagnosis of an incurable condition is made. The advanced directive allows for care and comfort for the patient, but withdraws permission for any "heroic" measures such as resuscitation or measures that would prolong the life of the patient such as intubation and ventilator support. An example of a living will or advanced directive can be found in the appendix. State laws pertaining to living wills vary. Prehospital care providers are urged to consult local and state EMS agencies pertaining to the acceptance of living wills in their states. See a sample of an advanced directive in the appendix.

Another form for healthcare direction is the DPOA for healthcare. The DPOA is more widely accepted and has more support in the law than the advanced directive. Also, the DPOA is easier to understand and more uniform in its structure.

The purpose of the DPOA is to allow another person to make healthcare decisions for the patient should the patient become unable to make those decisions. The person assigned to make healthcare decisions is known as the representative or agent. It is important for the patient to clearly express their wishes to the agent. Those wishes are then stated on the DPOA. In the event the initial representative is not available, a back-up agent should also be named on the document. A copy of the DPOA should be available at the patient's location. Copies should also be given to representatives, family members, the family lawyer, and the patient's physician. DPOAs may have a specified time limit or they may be in effect indefinitely. However, the patient may rescind the DPOA at any time as long as the patient is coherent and competent to make that decision. Prehospital care providers are urged to contact their local and state EMS agencies for more information regarding the use and validity of a DPOA in the prehospital setting. A sample of a DPOA is included in the appendix.

DO NOT RESUSCITATE (DNR)

Although the Patient Self-Determination Act did go a long way in securing a patient's right to accept or deny medical care, it was not clear how advanced directives would impact upon EMS. For many years, agencies had no clear guidelines, and some chose to ignore any advanced directive or self-generated DNR request. Terminally ill patients being transported to or from hospitals, skilled nursing facilities, or hospice had no guarantee that their requests for no resuscitation would be honored. To alleviate the confusion and establish clear standards pertaining to DNR orders, many states have enacted legislation or promulgated rules pertaining to DNR. These DNR orders allow the patient to decide in advance if CPR and life-prolonging therapy should be initiated. Although the laws and forms may vary between states, their intent is similar: Do Not Resuscitate means no chest compressions, artificial ventilation, defibrillation, intubation, or cardiac medications.

What DNR orders do not include is the withholding of care and comfort measures aimed at alleviating pain or suffering and making the patient more comfortable. Even in the presence of a DNR order, the patient is to receive care for shortness of breath, airway obstruction, bleeding, fractures, and other medical emergencies. However, if at any time breathing ceases, resuscitation efforts will be withheld.

The patient can override a DNR order at any time. For example, if the patient looks up and says, "Don't let me die," the DNR becomes invalid.

An example of a DNR form is included in the appendix.

KEY POINT

A patient who has a valid DNR can change their mind at any time and void the DNR. Voiding of the DNR does not have to be in writing.

In most cases, the DNR form spells out the procedures that are to be carried out. These procedures include:

- Posting or keeping the DNR in a readily accessible location. For patients in a hospital or skilled nursing facility, the DNR can be kept in the patient's records or in an envelope attached to the patient's bed. For a patient at home, the DNR can be kept inside the medicine cabinet or in a "Vial of Life" bottle inside the refrigerator. If the patient at home is in a hospital bed, the DNR can be kept in an envelope attached to the head of the bed. The form can also be posted on the door to the patient's bedroom or kept in the patient's wallet. Some states allow for medical ID necklaces and bracelets to state the DNR request.
- The prehospital care provider is to see the signed DNR. Some states allow the attending physician to verify the death and DNR or to write a DNR order in the patient's chart. A charted DNR is to be presented to the EMS crew on arrival at the scene of the call.
- Correctly identify the patient by driver's license, family identification, or other form of positive identification.
- If a family member is present and states that they would like resuscitation to be provided for the patient, prehospital care providers should make every effort to comply with the *patient's* wishes. If there is any doubt as to the patient's wishes, EMS crews should initiate CPR until the patient's wishes can be clarified.
- Document any patient contact on the patient care report. If required and available, attach a copy of the DNR to the patient care report.
- If appropriate and required by local policies and procedures, transport the patient to the emergency department or medical examiner's office.

The preceding information is intended only as a guide. Prehospital care providers should consult with their local and state EMS agencies for laws, rules, and forms that pertain to their specific state. There are still some legal gray areas that have yet to be addressed by the courts. For example, if the EMS crew is unaware of a DNR and resuscitates a patient, will they be held liable? If the DNR cannot be verified and CPR is provided, does the resuscitation pose liability for the prehospital care providers? The courts must answer these questions.

SUMMARY

Death is inevitable. Every person will eventually die. Prehospital care providers will be called to attend to the dying patient and perhaps provide care and comfort during the patient's final moments. This chapter discussed the dying patient, the concepts of hospice care, and changes to the body as it prepares to die. Additionally, this chapter presented information about the patient's right to decide if they will accept care and to what level.

The courts and the law have long upheld the concept that a patient has the right to decide the forms of healthcare they are willing to accept. The concept of expressed consent has been around for years. If a patient does not wish to receive CPR, how do they convey that message to healthcare workers? The Patient Self-Determination Act did clarify the issue and advanced directives were born.

However, do these same concepts apply to responding prehospital care providers? The Patient's Self-Determination Act answered many of those questions as they pertain to hospital care, yet prehospital care providers were in a quandary over increasingly used DNR orders. To alleviate the confusion, many states enacted laws and rules that clearly identified the prehospital care provider's role and responsibilities upon finding a DNR order. While the DNR laws do permit care, comfort, and other means of treatment for the patient, they do relieve EMS from the responsibility of performing CPR or providing resuscitation therapy to the dying patient against their wishes. This chapter described each of these legal concepts.

ON THE JOB

You respond to a call to an apartment building where you find a patient lying in a hospital bed located in the living room. The patient is a 67-year-old woman who appears to be emaciated. Family members tell you that the woman has terminal cancer and that she is a hospice patient. They hand you the woman's advanced directive and DNR order. You quickly assess the patient and find her responsive to physical stimulation only. Her breathing is shallow at six per minute and her pulse is 60 beats per minute and very weak. The woman is receiving oxygen via nasal cannula at 4 liters per minute. The family knows that the end is near and tells you that the woman has not eaten in 2 days. Do you transport the patient to the emergency department? Do you continue oxygen therapy en route to the hospital? Do you start IV therapy en route to the emergency department? If the patient stops breathing, what treatment would you provide?

13

Putting It All Together

OBJECTIVES

At the end of the chapter, the reader will be able to:

1 Demonstrate how to approach the patient with respect for the patient's age and status by addressing the patient using their surname.

2 Demonstrate how to protect the patient from extremes of the environment by covering the patient appropriately.

3 Demonstrate how to cover the patient with a loose blanket to prevent pain in or pressure on the feet.

4 Demonstrate how to pad tender areas of the body to alleviate pressure and reduce the chance of decubitus ulcers.

5 Explain why adhesive tape on the skin of the older adult may not be appropriate.

WORDS TO KNOW

Contracture   Permanent and abnormal position of a joint characterized by flexion of the joint. Seen in some patients after a stroke.

Methycillin-resistant staphylococcus aureus (MRSA)   Bacteria found in patients confined to hospitals or skilled nursing facilities. The bacteria do not respond to some antibiotics.

Nosocomial infection   Infection contracted while admitted to a hospital or skilled nursing facility.

Vancomycin-resistant enterococcus (VRE)   Bacteria normally found in the intestines that may be spread to other patients by healthcare workers. The bacteria do not respond to very powerful antibiotics.

From the start of this textbook through the previous chapter, we have discussed changes that take place in the body as we grow older and the conditions associated with those changes. Not only does the aging person experience physical changes, the person also experiences emotional changes. As we age, there is a tendency to develop chronic conditions that require lifelong attention, including the use of prescription medications. The end result of aging is an increased need for medical care. Prehospital care providers are a part of the medical care team that older adults rely upon when they become ill or injured. When responding to a medical complaint involving an elderly patient, prehospital care providers can use their knowledge about the effects of aging to provide better, more compassionate patient care. The purpose of this chapter is to "put it all together" with hints and tips to enable the prehospital care provider to give the precious gift of quality patient care while keeping in mind that patient care also means caring for the patient.

APPROACHING THE PATIENT

When initially approaching the elderly patient, use the patient's surname until instructed otherwise. Using the surname implies respect for the individual. For example, William Smith has called for help. Approaching the patient and saying, "Hi, Bill, how are you this morning?" is perhaps not the best introduction. Addressing the patient as Mr. Smith is more appropriate. If the patient replies, "Call me Bill," then use the patient's first name. The prehospital care provider may also ask, "Would it be OK if I called you Bill?"

When performing patient assessment, prehospital care providers often disrobe the patient. The concept of "strip and flip" often applies to trauma victims. Keeping the older adult covered as much as possible retains their dignity. If undressing the patient and partially exposing them is necessary, explain to the patient why it is necessary and ask for, but do not demand, their cooperation. If a patient is found in a public place and is in cardiac arrest where baring the chest is necessary to provide care, keep the patient's exposure to the public to a minimum.

It is sometimes difficult to understand the emotions, needs, and wants of another person. This can be especially true when caring for an older person. Research has shown that an individual can understand the emotions of another person half again their age. In other words, a 30-year-old person can understand the feelings of a 45-year-old person. Consider the barriers that exist when a

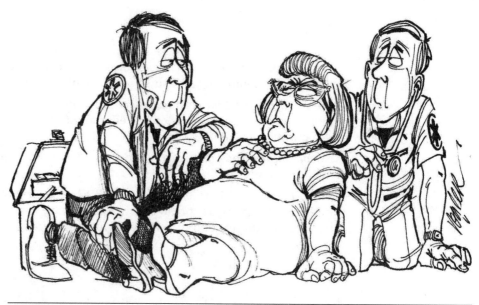

• FIGURE 13-1
"Ma'am, you can rest assured that neither my partner nor I will get any 'funny ideas' when treating you."
Source: Courtesy EES Publications.

20-year-old is conversing with a 90-year-old. The communications can be strained. To get a better understanding of the emotions of the older adult, use active listening and empathic listening techniques. In each of these techniques, the listener identifies the emotions behind what the other person is saying. These techniques take time and practice to perfect. For more information on empathic listening, refer to Stephen Covey's *Seven Habits of Highly Effective People.*

Do not be in a hurry. Most medical emergencies are over upon arrival of the EMS crew. Therefore, any need to rush or hurry is diminished by the time the prehospital care provider arrives on the scene. Older adults, even those who are mentally alert and oriented, may take a little longer to respond to questions or perform a task. Do not be impatient and do not expect the patient's responses to be immediate. Patients with dementia, delirium, stroke, or other conditions that affect their ability to process information may take even longer to respond.

Allow the patient to rest if they become fatigued. If the patient does not say that they are tired, ask, "Do you need to take a break?" Be perceptive of the patient's stamina and let the patient proceed at their own speed.

TRANSPORTING THE PATIENT

When transporting the patient, especially in a cold climate, be sure to protect the patient from the environment. Make sure the patient is dressed appropriately. In the event the patient is discharged from the hospital, ensure the patient has appropriate clothing for the trip home. Just like newborns, older adults lose heat from the head. In very cold temperatures, cover the patient's head to protect it from the environment and conserve body heat even if there is only a short distance between the building and the vehicle. To keep the patient warm on the gurney, wrap the blanket under the patient. This prevents a sudden, cold blast of air from getting under the blanket and chilling the patient.

When wrapping the blanket underneath the patient, be sure to keep the covering loose. Tight coverings, especially over the feet, can be painful. If the

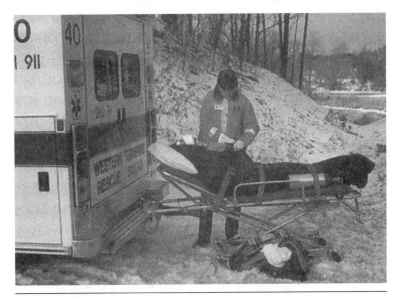

• FIGURE 13-2
In cold weather, protect the patient's head from heat loss and wrap blankets under patients.
Source: Courtesy Brady *Emergency Care* 8th ed., p. 677.

patient has arthritis or other deformity of the feet, pressure on the feet can be uncomfortable. Further, as was discussed in the section on decubitus ulcers, excess pressure can cause tissue damage to begin within a very short time. Finally, if the patient has existing bedsores on their heels or ankles, additional pressure created by tight blankets could worsen the injury.

Protect the patient from both heat and cold. Remove the patient from areas of temperature extremes as soon as possible. If the patient has collapsed on a hot asphalt surface such as a driveway, the heat will be transferred into the body. Similarly, if the patient has collapsed on an icy driveway or sidewalk, hypothermia can quickly develop.

Protect IV solutions from exposure to the cold. Cold IV solutions could induce or worsen hypothermia. Place the IV solution under the patient's pillow

• FIGURE 13-3
When wrapping blankets under patients or under the mattress, be sure the blankets over the patients feet are loose.
Source: Courtesy Brady *Prehospital Emergency Care* 5th ed., p. 732.

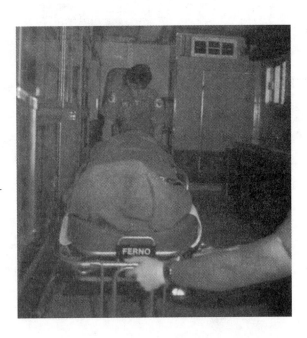

or wrap a towel or a washcloth around the bag when going outside in cold weather. Placing the bag under the patient's pillow will not only protect the solution from the cold, but also apply pressure to the bag and continue the flow of the solution. If possible, keep medications in a warm environment. If the vehicle is parked outside or in an unheated station, take the drug box inside the crew quarters in between calls to keep the medications from chilling. IV solutions can be kept warm inside a Styrofoam cooler that contains a sealed container of warm water or hot packs surrounded by bags of solution.

In addition to protecting the patient from the cold, protect the patient from accidental injury. If the patient is paralyzed or comatose, prevent the extremities from falling outside the gurney and striking a wall, table, or other piece of furniture. When placing the patient onto the gurney, be sure that the paralyzed arm or leg does not become trapped underneath the patient.

Patients with a prior history of stroke may have contractures of their affected arm. Pad the extremity when necessary and protect it from rubbing against other areas of the body, especially areas where bony prominences are likely to create pressure. The shearing forces can begin the process of skin deterioration that lead to decubitus ulcers.

Keep the heels and ankles away from the metal frame and pad those areas that could be exposed to pressure. Patients with bedsores should have the affected area padded. If the patient is placed in a left, lateral recumbent position, place a pillow between the patient's legs to reduce pressure from the bones of the knee.

One of the principles of medical care is "First, do no harm." This principle applies to all aspects of medical care including prehospital treatment. Knowing that an older person's skin may be fragile, the prehospital care provider should avoid using adhesive tape when securing a dressing or bandage to the skin. Removing adhesive tape from the skin can cause the skin to tear. Also, be careful with the gurney straps. The rough edges of the straps can abrade the older adult's skin.

When applying stretcher straps, especially over the older adult, do not secure any strap below the knees. Also, do not apply the strap to soft tissue or an area of the body that is not supported or protected by bone, that is, the abdomen.

Placing and securing a strap below the knee puts downward pressure on the shin. Without padding, the pressure can decrease circulation to the area and tissue deterioration may ensue. Also, placing a strap below the knee stresses the knee by putting backward pressure on the joint. This could cause a patient with degenerative joint disease or arthritis of the knee to experience severe pain.

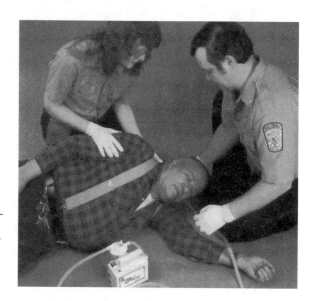

• FIGURE 13-4
Patient in left, lateral recumbent position.

Source: Courtesy Brady *Emergency Care,* p. 804.

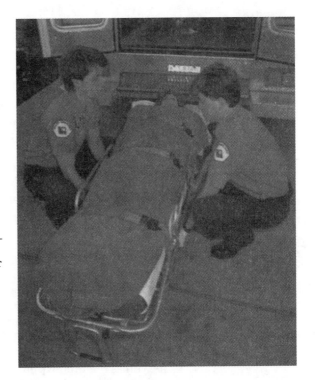

• FIGURE 13-5
Straps should be placed over bony areas such as across the chest, pelvis, and thigh. Do not place straps below the knees.

Source: Courtesy Brady *Prehospital Emergency Care* 5th ed., p. 732.

Finally, straps over soft tissue such as the abdomen do not support or restrain the patient adequately. In the event of an accident, the straps can cause severe damage to the abdominal organs.

Once the patient is placed inside the ambulance, switch to humidified oxygen for the trip to the hospital. Dry gas tends to dry the airways and mucus. This can interfere with the patient's ability to clear secretions from the airways.

Beware the nosocomial infection. Patients who are confined to a hospital or skilled nursing facility may have an infection that is easily spread to other patients. An infection that is contracted while hospitalized or admitted to a skilled nursing facility is called a nosocomial infection. Healthcare workers who contact the infectious patient, then provide care to subsequent patients without disinfecting themselves spread these infections among patients.

Some of the nosocomial infections are extremely difficult to combat. Infections such as methycillin-resistant staphylococcus aureus (MRSA) and vancomycin-resistant enterococcus (VRE) do not respond to commonly available antibiotics. Other infections such as pneumonia, influenza, and scabies, while easily treated, can infect the EMS crew as well as other patients and healthcare workers if precautions are not taken. Be sure to use universal precautions such as gloves, as well as goggles, mask, and gown where appropriate. Always wash your hands and all exposed skin after every patient contact.

Finally, when preparing to transport the patient and leaving the home, if the patient says, "Wait a moment. I want to take one last look around. I am not coming back," the prehospital care provider should grant the patient's request. Patients often know when the end is near and allowing them time to say good-bye is an added plus in caring for and about the patient.

HOW DO YOU FEEL?

This book has approached caring for the elderly patient from a prehospital care provider perspective. Eventually, the reader of this book, you, will be older or, by some descriptions, old. The aging process is slow and insidious. Without realizing it, the gray hair appears, the arcus senilis develops, and things start to slow down. Middle age comes on suddenly and gradually. We all get old—all while we were too busy living and making a living to notice. The children grow up quickly and develop lives of their own. Soon, you start hearing the word "Grandpa" or "Grandma," and suddenly realize that child is talking to *you*.

Perhaps it might be wise to assess your own feelings about aging, chronic illness, death, and dying. A negative attitude toward aging could reflect on the quality of care. It is important to acknowledge your own feelings about getting older and deal with any hostilities you may uncover. Keep in mind that you could be in the nursing home one day and need the help of those younger, prehospital care providers.

None of us want to grow old, but we do, and we need to examine our feelings about aging.

SUMMARY

The older patient has needs that are similar to yet different from those of a younger adult. The body is less flexible and more prone to illness and injury. The older adult can become hypothermic or overheated very quickly, even in the absence of temperature extremes. This chapter has mentioned a few things that will make caring for the elderly patient a bit less traumatic for the patient as well as the prehospital care provider. At times, some of the tried and true procedures that work well in the younger adult may have to be dismissed to provide proper care for the older patient. If in doubt about any procedure, ask! No, not the physician on the radio or other crew members. Ask the patient! And, listen to patient's needs. After all, the most important word in the phrase "patient care" is care.

Appendix

In various chapters of the text, there have been references to finding additional information in the appendix. The nature of an appendix is to contain items that are frequently used or referenced in an easy-to-find location. This appendix includes several valuable items that can be used by EMS agencies in a variety of ways:

- State Agencies on Aging—an alphabetical list of each state's department that is responsible for assisting the elderly.
- National Institute of Health Stroke Scale—an 11-point score that is used when accessing a patient suspected of having a stroke.
- Check for Safety—a checklist for home safety developed by the CDC's National Center for Injury Prevention and Control (NCIPC). This checklist can be copied from this appendix or downloaded from the NCIPC Web site at www.cdc.gov/ncipc. This checklist is an excellent tool for those EMS agencies that want to provide an in-home safety assessment for the seniors in the community.
- Do Not Resuscitate, Advanced Directive, and Durable Power of Attorney forms—samples of the forms from various states including Texas, California, Tennessee, West Virginia, and Florida are included to give examples of the types of forms encountered in the field.

Use this appendix as a reference while reading the text and later as a resource to assist the elderly in the community.

State Agencies on Aging

Alabama
Department of Senior Services
RSA Plaza. Suite 470
770 Washington Ave.
Montgomery, AL 36130
(334) 242-5743   (877) 425-2243

Alaska
Commission on Aging
Division of Senior Services
PO Box 110209
Juneau, AK 99811-0209
(907) 465-3250

Arizona
Aging and Adult Administration
1789 West Jefferson
Site Code 950A
Phoenix, AZ 85007
(602) 542-4446

Arkansas
Division of Aging and Adult
  Services
PO Box 1437, Slot 1412
1417 Donaghey Plaza South
Little Rock, AR 72203-1437
(501) 682-2441

California
Department of Aging
1600 K Street
Sacramento, CA 95814
(916) 322-3887   (800) 510-2020

Colorado
Department of Aging and Adult
  Services
110 16th Street, 2nd Floor
Denver, CO 80203
(303) 620-4147

Connecticut
Department of Social Services
Division of Elderly Services
25 Sigourney Street, 10th Floor
Hartford, CT 06106-5033
(203) 424-5277

Delaware
Division of Services for Aging
  and Adults with Physical
  Disabilities
1901 North DuPont Highway
New Castle: DE 19720
(302) 577-4791   (800) 223-9074

District of Columbia
Office on Aging
441 4th Street NW
Suite 900 South
Washington, DC 20001
(202) 724-5622

Florida
Department of Elder Affairs
4040 Esplanade Way Ste. 152
Tallahassee, FL 32399-0700
(850) 414-2000   (800) 963-5337

Georgia
Division of Aging Services
2 Peachtree Street NW Ste. 36-385
Atlanta, GA 30303-3142
(404) 657-5319

Hawaii
Executive Office on Aging
250 South Hotel Street Ste. 109
Honolulu, HI 96813-2813
(808) 586-0185

Idaho
State Commission on Aging
3380 Americana Terrace Ste. 20
PO Box 83720
Boise, ID 83706
(208) 334-3833

Illinois
Department on Aging
421 East Capitol Ave. Ste. 100
Springfield, IL 62701-1789
(217) 785-2870

Indiana
Bureau of Aging and In-Home
  Services
402 West Washington Street
PO Box 7083
Indianapolis, IN 46207-7083
(317) 232-7020   (800) 545-7763

Iowa
Department of Elder Affairs
200 Tenth Street Ste. 300
Des Moines, IA 50309-3609
(515) 281-5187

Kansas
Department on Aging
New England Building
503 S. Kansas Ave.
Topeka, KS 66603-3404
(913) 296-4986   (800) 432-3535

Kentucky
Office of Aging Services
275 East Main Street 5W-A
Frankfort, KY 40621
(502) 564-6930

Louisiana
Governor's Office of Elderly
  Affairs
412 North 4th Street
PO Box 80374
Baton Rouge, LA 70898-0374
(225) 925-1700

Maine
Bureau of Elder and Adult
  Services
35 Anthony Ave.
11 State House Station
Augusta, ME 04333-0011
(207) 624-5335

Maryland
Department of Aging
301 West Preston Street 10th Floor
Baltimore, MD 21201-2374
(410) 767-1100

Massachusetts
Executive Office of Elder Affairs
One Ashburton Place 5th Floor
Boston, MA 02108
(617) 727-7750   (800) 882-2003

Michigan
Office of Services to the Aging
611 West Ottawa
PO Box 30676
Lansing, MI 48909-8176
(517) 373-8230

Minnesota
Board on Aging
444 Lafayette Road
St. Paul, MN 55155-3843
(612) 296-2770   (800) 333-2433

Mississippi
Council on Aging
750 State Street
Jackson, MS 39202
(601) 359-4929   (800) 948-3090

Missouri
Division on Aging
615 Howerton Court
PO Box 1337
Jefferson City, MO 65102-1337
(573) 751-3082   (800) 235-5503

Montana
Governor's Office on Aging
PO Box 8005
Helena, MT 59604-8005
(406) 444-7787   (800) 332-2272

Nebraska
Division on Aging
1342 M Street
PO Box 95044
Lincoln, NE 68509-5044
(402) 471-2307   (800) 942-7830

Nevada
Aging Services Division
340 North 11th Street Ste. 303
Las Vegas, NV 89101
(702) 486-3545

New Hampshire
Division of Elderly and Adult
  Services
129 Pleasant Street
Concord, NH 03301-3857
(603) 271-4680   (800) 351-1888

New Jersey
Department of Health and Senior
  Services
Quaker Bridge Plaza
Quaker Bridge Road
PO Box 807
Trenton, NJ 08625-0807
(609) 588-3141   (800) 792-8820

New Mexico
State Agency on Aging
La Villa Rivera Building, Ground
  Floor
228 East Palace Avenue
Santa Fe, NM 87501
(505) 827-7640   (800) 432-2080

New York
State Office for the Aging
Agency Building 2
Albany, NY 12223-1251
(518) 474-5731   (800) 342-9871

North Carolina
Division of Aging
693 Palmer Drive
CB 29531
Raleigh, NC 27626-0531
(919) 733-3983   (800) 662-7030

North Dakota
Aging Services Division
600 South 2nd Street Ste. 1C
Bismarck, ND 58504-5279
(701) 328-8910   (800) 451-8693

Ohio
Department of Aging
50 West Broad Street 9th Floor
Columbus, OH 43215-3363
(614) 466-5500

Oklahoma
Aging Services Division
312 Northeast 28th Street
PO Box 25352
Oklahoma City, OK 73112
(405) 521-2327

Oregon
Senior and Disabled Services
500 Summer Street NE 2nd Floor
Salem, OR 97310-1015
(503) 945-5811   (800) 282-8096

Pennsylvania
Department of Aging
400 Market Street 6th Floor
Harrisburg, PA 17101-2301
(717) 783-3126

Rhode Island
Department of Elderly Affairs
160 Pine Street
Providence, RI 02903-3708
(401) 222-2894 ext. 301
(800) 322-2880

South Carolina
Office on Aging
202 Arbor Lake Drive Ste. 301
PO Box 8206
Columbia, SC 29202
(803) 253-4173   (800) 868-9095

South Dakota
Office of Adult Services and Aging
700 Governors Drive
Pierre, SD 57501-2291
(605) 773-3656

Tennessee
Commission on Aging
Andrew Jackson Building
500 Deaderick Street 9th Floor
Nashville, TN 37243-0860
(615) 741-2056

Texas
Department on Aging
4900 North Lamar 4th Floor
PO Box 12786 Capitol Station
Austin, TX 78711
(512) 424-6840

Utah
Aging Services
120 North 200 West Room 401
Box 45500
Salt Lake City, UT 84103
(801) 538-3910

Vermont
Department of Aging and
   Disabilities
Waterbury Complex
103 South Main Street
Waterbury, VT 05671
(802) 241-2325

Virginia
Department for the Aging
1600 Forest Ave. Ste. 102
Richmond, VA 23229
(804) 662-9333   (800) 662-9354

Washington
Aging and Adult Services
Administration
PO Box 45600
Olympia, WA 98504-5600
(360) 493-2500

West Virginia
Bureau of Senior Services
Holly Grove, Bldg 10
1900 Kanawha Boulevard East
Charleston, WV 25305-0160
(304) 558-3317   (877) 987-4463

Wisconsin
Bureau on Aging
217 South Hamilton Street
Ste. 300
Madison, WI 53703
(608) 266-2536

Wyoming
Division on Aging
Hathaway Building
2300 Capital Avenue Room 139
Cheyenne, WY 82002-0480
(307) 777-7986   (800) 442-2766

National Institute of Health Stroke Scale

1a. Level of Consciousness
  0 Alert
  1 Not alert; arousable with minimal stimulation
  2 Not alert; requires repeated stimulation to attend
  3 Coma

1b. Ask patient the month and their age
  0 Answers both correctly
  1 Answers one correctly
  2 Answers both incorrectly

1c. Ask patient to open and close eyes
  0 Obeys both correctly
  1 Obeys one correctly
  2 Obeys both incorrect

2. Best gaze (only horizontal eye movement)
  0 Normal
  1 Partial gaze palsy
  2 Forced deviation

3. Visual field testing
  0 No visual field loss
  1 Partial hemianopia (loss of one-half of vision)
  2 Complete hemianopia (loss of one-half of vision)

4. Facial paresis (Ask patient to show symmetrical movement—show teeth or raise eyebrows and close eyes tightly)
  0 Normal
  1 Minor paralysis (asymmetry on smiling)
  2 Partial paralysis (near total paralysis of lower face)
  3 Complete paralysis of one or both sides (absence of facial movement)

5. Motor function—arm (right and left): Extends arm 45 or 90 degrees for 10 seconds without drift
  0 Normal
  1 Drift
  2 Some effort against gravity
  3 No effort against gravity
  4 No movement
  9 Untestable—joint fused or limb amputated

6. Motor function—leg (right and left): Hold leg in 30 degrees position for 5 seconds
  0 Normal
  1 Drift
  2 Some effort against gravity
  3 No effort against gravity
  4 No movement
  9 Untestable—joint fused or limb amputated

7. Limb ataxia
  0 No ataxia
  1 Present in one limb
  2 Present in two limbs

8. Sensory—pinprick to tests arms, legs, trunk, and face; compare side to side
  0 Normal
  1 Mild to moderate decrease in sensation
  2 Severe to total sensory loss

9. Best language—describe picture, name items, read sentences
  0 No aphasia
  1 Mild to moderate aphasia

2 Severe aphasia
3 Mute

10. Dysarthria—read several words
   0 Normal articulation
   1 Mild to moderate slurring of words
   2 Near unintelligible or unable to speak
   9 Intubated or other physical barrier

11. Extinction and inattention—able to recognize sensory stimulation bilaterally
   0 Normal
   1 Inattention or extinction to bilateral simultaneous stimulation in one sensory modality
   2 Severe hemi-inattention or hemi-inattention to more than one sensory modality

Check For Safety

A Home Fall Prevention Checklist for Older Adults

This checklist is a publication of the National Center for Injury Prevention and Control of the Centers for Disease Control and Prevention.

Centers for Disease Control and Prevention
Jeffrey P. Koplan, MD, MPH, Director

National Center for Injury Prevention and Control
Mark L. Rosenberg, MD, MPP, Director

Division of Unintentional Injury Prevention
Christine M. Branche, PhD, Director

Authors
Judy A. Stevens, PhD
Sarah J. Olson, MS, CHES

Production services were provided by the staff of the Office of Health Communications, National Center for Injury Prevention and Control.

October 1999

FALLS AT HOME

Each year, thousands of older Americans fall at home. Many of them are seriously injured, and some are disabled. In 1996, more than 8,500 people over age 65 died because of falls.

Falls are often due to hazards that are easy to overlook but easy to fix. This checklist will help you find and fix those hazards in your home.

The checklist asks about hazards found in each room of your home. For each hazard, the checklist tells you how to fix the problem. At the end of the checklist, you will find other tips for preventing falls.

FLOORS

Look at the floor in each room.

Q. When you walk through a room, do you have to walk around furniture?
   ❏ Ask someone to move the furniture so your path is clear.

Q. Do you have throw rugs on the floor?
   ❏ Remove the rugs or use double-sided tape or a non-slip backing so the rugs won't slip.

Q. Are papers, magazines, books, shoes, boxes, blankets, towels, or other objects on the floor?
   ❏ Pick up things that are on the floor. Always keep objects off the floor.

Q. Do you have to walk over or around cords or wires (like cords from lamps, extension cords, or telephone cords)?
   ❏ Coil or tape cords and wires next to the wall so you can't trip over them. Have an electrician put in another outlet.

STAIRS AND STEPS

Look at the stairs you use both inside and outside your home.

Q. Are papers, shoes, books, or other objects on the stairs?
- ❏ Pick up things on the stairs. Always keep objects off the stairs.

Q. Are some steps broken or uneven?
- ❏ Fix loose or uneven steps.

Q. Are you missing a light over the stairway?
- ❏ Have a maintenance person or an electrician put in an overhead light at the top and bottom of the stairs.

Q. Has the stairway light bulb burned out?
- ❏ Have a friend or family member change the light bulb.

Q. Do you have only one light switch for your stairs (only at the top or at the bottom of the stairs)?
- ❏ Have a maintenance person or an electrician put in a light switch at the top and bottom of the stairs. You can get light switches that glow.

Q. Are the handrails loose or broken? Is there a handrail on only one side of the stairs?
- ❏ Fix loose handrails or put in new ones. Make sure handrails are on both sides of the stairs and are as long as the stairs.

Q. Is the carpet on the steps loose or torn?
- ❏ Make sure the carpet is firmly attached to every step or remove the carpet and attach non-slip rubber treads on the stairs.

KITCHEN

Look at your kitchen and eating area.

Q. Are the things you use often on high shelves?
- ❏ Move items in your cabinets. Keep things you use often on the lower shelves (about waist high).

Q. Is your step stool unsteady?
- ❏ Get a new, steady step stool with a bar to hold on to. Never use a chair as a step stool.

BEDROOMS

Look at all your bedrooms.

Q. Is the light near the bed hard to reach?
- ❏ Place a lamp close to the bed where it is easy to reach.

Q. Is the path from your bed to the bathroom dark?
- ❏ Put in a night-light so you can see where you're walking. Some night-lights go on by themselves after dark.

BATHROOMS

Look at all your bathrooms.

Q. Is the tub or shower floor slippery?
- ❏ Put a non-slip rubber mat or self-stick strips on the floor of the tub or shower.

Q. Do you have some support when you get in and out of the tub or up from the toilet?

- ❏ Have a maintenance person or a carpenter put in a grab bar inside the tub and next to the toilet.

OTHER THINGS YOU CAN DO TO PREVENT FALLS

- ❏ Exercise regularly. Exercise makes you stronger and improves your balance and coordination.
- ❏ Have your doctor or pharmacist look at all the medicines you take, even over-the-counter medicines. Some medicines can make you sleepy or dizzy.
- ❏ Have your vision checked at least once a year by an eye doctor. Poor vision can increase risk of falling.
- ❏ Get up slowly after you sit or lie down.
- ❏ Wear sturdy shoes with thin, non-slip soles. Avoid slippers and running shoes with thick soles.
- ❏ Improve the lighting in your home. Use brighter light bulbs (at least 60 watts). Use lamp shades or frosted bulbs to reduce glare.
- ❏ Use reflecting tape at the top and bottom of the stairs so you can see them better.
- ❏ Paint doorsills a different color to prevent tripping.

OTHER SAFETY TIPS

- ❏ Keep emergency numbers in large print near each phone.
- ❏ Put a phone near the floor in case you fall and can't get up.
- ❏ Think about wearing an alarm device that will bring help in case you fall and can't get up.

For more information contact:

The National Center for Injury Prevention and Control
Division of Unintentional Injury Prevention
4770 Buford Highway, NE, Mailstop K-63
Atlanta, GA 30341

www.cdc.gov/ncipc

www.cdc.gov/safeusa

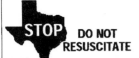

TEXAS DEPARTMENT OF HEALTH STANDARD
OUT-OF-HOSPITAL DO-NOT-RESUSCITATE ORDER

STOP DO NOT RESUSCITATE

This document becomes effective immediately on the date of execution.
It remains in effect until the death of the patient or the document is revoked.

1. _____ Date of Birth: _____ Male/Female (Circle One)

    Patient's full legal name — printed or typed

2. COMPLETE <u>ONE</u> OF THE FOLLOWING THREE BOXES: A, B, OR C.

A. **Patient's Statement:** I, the undersigned, am capable of making an informed decision regarding the withholding or withdrawing of CPR, including the treatments listed below, and I direct that none of the following resuscitation measures be initiated or continued. **Cardiopulmonary resuscitation (CPR), Transcutaneous Cardiac Pacing, Defibrillation, Advanced Airway Management, Artificial Ventilation**
I understand that I will be given comfort measures as needed. I understand that I may revoke this order at any time.

_____ _____ _____
Signature   Date   Printed or Typed Name

B. **Only use this box if the order is being completed by a person acting on behalf of a patient who is incompetent or otherwise unable to make his or her wishes known**

I am the patient's: ☐ legal guardian; ☐ agent under Medical Power of Attorney; ☐ managing conservator; ☐ Qualified Relative (see back); or parent of a minor child **AND:**

☐ I attest to issuance of an Out-of-Hospital DNR by the patient by nonwritten means of communication; **OR**
☐ I am acting under the guidance of a prior Directive to Physicians; **OR**
☐ I am acting upon the known values and desires of the patient; **OR**
☐ I am acting in the patient's best interest based upon the guidance given by the patient's physician.
I direct that none of the following resuscitation measures be initiated or continued; Cardiopulmonary resuscitation (CPR), Transcutaneous Cardiac Pacing, Defibrillation, Advanced Airway Management, Artificial Ventilation on behalf of the patient.

_____ _____ _____
Signature   Date   Printed or Typed Name

• FIGURE A-1

Texas Department of Health standard out-of-hospital do-not-resuscitate order.

Source: www.tdh.state.tx.us/hcqs/ems/dnrhome.htm.

FLORIDA
DO NOT RESUSCITATE ORDER
(Please use ink)

EMS

Patient's Full Legal Name _____

               (Print or Type Name)   (Date)

PATIENT'S STATEMENT

Based upon informed consent, I, the undersigned, hereby direct that CPR be withheld or withdrawn.
(If not signed by patient, check applicable box):
☐ Surrogate   ☐ Proxy (both as defined in Chapter 765, F.S.)
☐ Court appointed guardian   ☐ Durable power of attorney (pursuant to Chapter 709, F.S.)

_____ _____
(Applicable Signature)   (Print or Type Name)

PHYSICIAN'S STATEMENT

• FIGURE A-2

Florida do not resuscitate order.

Source: www.doh.state.fl.us/ems/1General/6Resuscitate/Dnro.htm.

Directive to Physicians and Family or Surrogates

Advance Directives Act (see '166.033, Health and Safety Code)

This is an important legal document known as an Advance Directive. It is designed to help you communicate your wishes about medical treatment at some time in the future when you are unable to make your wishes known because of illness or injury. These wishes are usually based on personal values. In particular, you may want to consider what burdens or hardships of treatment you would be willing to accept for a particular amount of benefit obtained if you were seriously ill.

You are encouraged to discuss your values and wishes with your family or chosen spokesperson, as well as your physician. Your physician, other health care provider, or medical institution may provide you with various resources to assist you in completing your advance directive. Brief definitions are listed below and may aid you in your discussions and advance planning. Initial the treatment choices that best reflect your personal preferences. Provide a copy of your directive to your physician, usual hospital, and family or spokesperson. Consider a periodic review of the document. By periodic review, you can best assure that the directive reflects your preferences.

In addition to this advance directive, Texas law provides for two other types of directives that can be important during a serious illness. These are the Medical Power of Attorney and the Out-of-Hospital Do-Not-Resuscitate Order. You may wish to discuss these with your physician, family, hospital representative, or other advisers. You may also wish to complete a directive related to the donation of organs and tissues.

Directive

I, _____, recognize that the best health care is based upon a partnership of trust and communication with my physician. My physician and I will make health care decisions together as long as I am of sound mind and able to make my wishes known. If there comes a time that I am unable to make medical decisions about myself because of illness or injury, I direct that the following treatment preferences be honored:

• FIGURE A-3

Directive to physicians and family or surrogates.
Source: ltc/dhs.tx.us/policy/advanced/livgwill.htm.

Medical Power Of Attorney

Advance Directives Act (see '166.164, Health and Safety Code)

Designation of Health Care Agent:

I, _____ (insert your name) appoint:

Name: _____

Address: _____

_____ Phone: _____
as my agent to make any and all health care decisions for me, except to the extent I state otherwise in this document. This medical power of attorney takes effect if I become unable to make my own health care decisions and this fact is certified in writing by my physician.

Limitations On The Decision Making Authority Of My Agent Are As Follows:

_____

_____

Designation of an Alternate Agent:
(You are not required to designate an alternate agent but you may do so. An alternate agent may make the same health care decisions as the designated agent if the designated agent is unable or unwilling to act as your agent. If the agent designated is your spouse, the designation is automatically revoked by law if your marriage is dissolved.)

If the person designated as my agent is unable or unwilling to make health care decisions for me, I designate the following person(s), to serve as my agent to make health care decisions for me as authorized by this document, who serve in the following order:

• FIGURE A-4

Medical power of attorney.
Source: ltc/dhs.state.tx.us/policy/advance/medpoa2.htm.

Index